Lifeblood

Also by Mina Holland
The Edible Atlas
Mamma

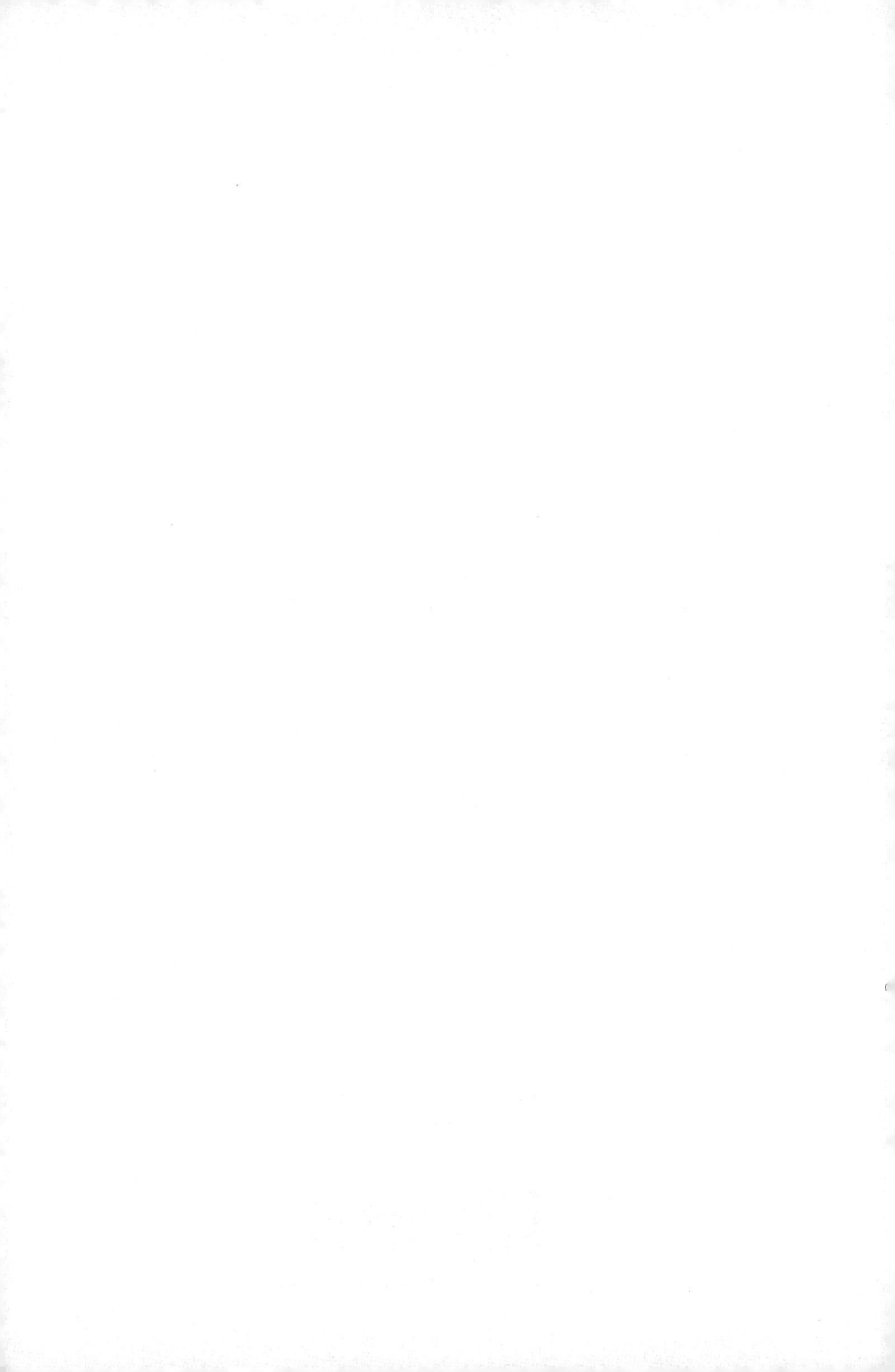

Lifeblood
A Mother in Search of Hope

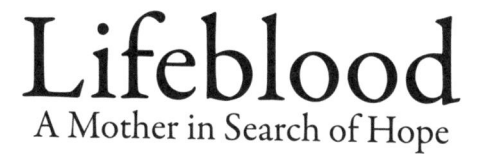

Mina Holland

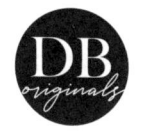

First published in the United Kingdom in 2025 by
Daunt Books
83 Marylebone High Street
London W1U 4QW
publishing@dauntbooks.co.uk

1

Copyright © Mina Holland, 2025

The right of Mina Holland to be identified as author of
this work has been asserted by her in accordance with the
Copyright, Designs and Patents Act 1988

All rights reserved. No part of this publication may be
reproduced, stored in a retrieval system, copied or transmitted,
in any form or by any means without the prior written
permission from Daunt Books, nor be otherwise circulated
in any form of binding or cover other than that in which it is
published and without a similar condition being imposed on
the subsequent purchaser

Extract from Labi Siffre's 'Blood on the Page' is from *Blood on the Page*
(Xavier Books) and used with the kind permission of Labi Siffre

Extract from 'Morning Song' by Sylvia Plath is from her *Collected
Poems* used with the kind permission of Faber & Faber

A CIP catalogue record for this title is available from the British Library

ISBN 978-1-917092-08-1

Typeset by Marsha Swan

Printed and bound by Bell and Bain Ltd., Glasgow

www.dauntbookspublishing.co.uk

*For Freddie, Vida and Gabriel,
and for the NHS*

And when the blood flows
Fill your pen from the wound
And write
LABI SIFFRE, 'Blood on the Page'

Prologue

Her name means life. Vida. A name as basic, you could say, as Baby or Human.

She had it before she was born – not that we used it. Vida was always a quiet understanding between us, the name that this baby, this life, would go by once she'd made her appearance.

Bleary eyed on her first night in the world – our fifth in hospital – we started to use it tentatively between hushes. 'Vida ... Vida', the only word we could muster for the creature wrapped in blankets, with its imp-like face and sweep of russet-brown hair.

My husband Freddie and I arrived at her name from different routes. I loved the word: its meaning, which captured the very essence of what we had made; its sound: two syllables, up-down; and its look: the peaceful V, and a happy balance of vowels and consonants. Small and powerful.

Freddie came to it via a favourite song of his mum's, 'Gracias a la Vida', covered by the Argentine singer Mercedes Sosa. This tune and its message had punctuated many moments in his childhood: car journeys, weekend breakfasts, colouring at the kitchen table. 'Thanks to life, which has given me so much,' Sosa sings. It is a song about laughter and tears, bliss and brokenness. New motherhood would come to show me the extent to which these extremes can co-exist; in making life, I broke and was remade.

Four months after that first night in hospital, Vida was diagnosed with a life-limiting blood disorder. So began a routine of complicated treatments: blood transfusions, toxic medications, innumerable interventions. Life as we knew it was punctured by cannula needles and transfused with a singular anxiety.

Before, I didn't see that the song's two materials, bliss and brokenness, are together emblematic of life itself. Nor that, no matter the breakage, bliss can prevail.

There was a time when I thought giving Vida this name had been inviting fate. Like a clumsy Grace or a miserable Felicity.

Few things make less sense than a sick child. I spent months looking for meaning, and I found no answers. At times it felt like prolonged vertigo, tussling with the implications of a disease that's mostly invisible in a child who was so – well, so *well*, most of the time, but whose very existence hung on other people's kindness. 'Packed red blood cells', as doctors call the plump bags of scarlet taken from the veins of blood donors. Bags which seem incongruously small when you consider the force of their contents.

Other people's blood became a fuel for my family. For a long time I struggled with nurses' references to 'topping her up', as though she were pulling into a petrol station. Every three weeks we returned. Haematologists have calculated that it takes about this long for patients with red-cell disorders – conditions affecting the blood cells which carry oxygen around the body with a protein called haemoglobin – to start running low. Without a transfusion, a baby like Vida will become symptomatic – unable to settle, lacking appetite, listless, distressed. These refuels, then, are an obligatory road tax for families like ours.

But are we unlucky? Nowadays, I look upon the contents of those blood bags reverentially, for I know they carry an elixir that has supported Vida's life.

Her name has helped me, too; maybe it will also help her one day. I hope she feels the strength of those letters we chose for her. A name, and a word, that holds up the power of her body, which fights a muddled message from a faulty gene and keeps going. It says, *I am here, and I am life*.

Lifeblood. One word, two definitions.

Blood, to Vida: *The blood, as being necessary to life*.

My children, to me: *The indispensable factor or influence that gives something its strength and vitality*.

Before

The morning we found out I was pregnant was unusual. It's not every day that I get a positive pregnancy test. Nor that I go kayaking.

It was June 2018 and we were visiting my husband Freddie's uncle in Cornwall. We got up at 5 a.m. so that, as the sun came up, we would already be on the Camel – a capillary of a river where we were staying near Wadebridge, which winds and widens into a vein that pulses out to sea at Padstow. It was a still and bright morning.

Something that day felt different to the times before, even though I couldn't put my finger on what. When I sat down to take the test, I was quietly confident. It was one of the electronic ones where the result flashes up before your eyes, then disappears briefly before flashing up again. 'Pregnant,' it said,

'1–2 weeks.' Was I seeing it correctly? But there it was again. And again.

'Pregnant,' I repeated, softly, laughing. Suddenly everything felt kinetic, electric. Newly energetic. 'Freddie!'

He rushed in, I held up the test. He let out a gasp and we hugged, too overcome to speak. Uncle Simon revved his car's engine in the driveway, anxious to catch that magical hour on the river. I finished my cup of tea, tied up my hair, grabbed my phone – ordinary actions that had already acquired a new dimension. I felt changed entirely.

On the river, Fred and I boarded a shared kayak that wobbled at the gentle current's every whim: nature's subject, and a metaphor for what was to come. Not that things seemed remotely precarious then. I felt strong, bolstered by the life I was growing. I glowed with its novelty, basked in its secrecy, and radiated a light mirrored by the dawn's sharp rays shooting through reeds.

It had been a long six months. Once we decided to start trying for a baby, I assumed it would be quick. I'd had an unplanned pregnancy in the past, and a 1990s sex education had instilled in me the idea that getting knocked up would be easy. At school, someone knew someone who'd got pregnant from a toilet seat, and I remember reading an older girl's magazine on the school coach, rapt over an article about a seventeen-year-old who'd gone to the loo and emerged with a baby, having had no idea she was pregnant at all. Rooted deep in my unconscious was the assumption that baby-making was simple, that eggs are sperm magnets.

Like many millennials with a similar background to mine, I'd grown up to believe that most of what I wanted was attainable. My privilege offered me opportunities and the confidence and work ethic to seize them, so that even though I didn't consider myself especially talented, things had a habit of falling into place. At university and in an unhappy relationship, I decided to apply to study abroad in America and sailed into my campus of choice. As a student, I decided I wanted to work in advertising and got onto a highly competitive grad scheme. As a graduate, I decided I didn't like advertising and wanted to be a food writer, a field in which only a handful of jobs exist, yet somehow bagged a book deal and a job at the *Guardian* within a year of leaving my previous career. Call it flukey, call it the ease of privilege, but in this way, my life had trundled along to a metronome of good fortune.

Trying for a baby would be the same story – right? Have sex, get pregnant. We'd just got married and lived a life I now remember in sepia. We'd done up a small flat in south-east London in thrifty good taste (raw plaster walls, a plywood kitchen, optimal storage so everything could be neatly put away) and we loved our jobs – Freddie is a composer, I'm a journalist, and at the time worked on the *Guardian*'s food desk part-time, with freelance writing on the side.

My first maternal stirrings were abated by a dog. I wanted one urgently and was broody for velvety snouts and mole-soft ears. After some resistance and a weekend looking after our friends' whippet, Freddie conceded to getting one of our own. From the moment Ernie arrived, lanky and gunmetal-grey, he embodied the battleground of our relationship. I wanted him on the sofa, Freddie didn't. Civilised evenings in front of the TV were peppered with kibble farts – we suspected he was wheat intolerant. He was accident prone. He was dumped by his dog walker when he bit another dog on her watch. And we never quite knew (and still don't) when he might take a dislike to a dog for whom he really wasn't a match – Rottweilers, Dobermans, Alsatians (you have to admire his chutzpah). My love for the dog was unconditional, and Freddie grudgingly developed feelings for him. It was all very *Beethoven*.

When I didn't get pregnant as easily as I'd imagined, I leant on my old chums graft and capitalism to help me reach my goal. I learnt my body's cues, downloaded menstrual-tracking apps, bought ovulation sticks and fertility lubricants. Still nothing. I became frenzied. A bad habit of consulting the internet set in. I became an avid Mumsnet user, where other people's stories ran the gamut of comforting to terrifying, a lit match to the wick of my uneasy hope for a baby. I was soon fluent in its acronyms – TTC (trying to conceive), DTD (do the deed, have sex), BD (baby dance, another one for DTD) – and a voyeur on its message boards, where I'd look for the testimonies of other women with symptoms similar to my own. Fast-growing fingernails, metallic mouth taste, cravings for malt loaf. Was I pregnant?

Try not to think about it went the advice, just enjoy having sex. Put your legs in the air afterwards, suggested my mum, making me immediately regret confiding in her. I yo-yoed between treating my body like a temple and hoovering up the wine and cheese I wouldn't be allowed if and when I got pregnant. For six months, failure greeted me every month in the form of a period.

When we got the positive test in Cornwall, our happiness about impending parenthood was quickly followed by huge relief that we could go to bed at night just to go to sleep. It was also permission to start preparing to become parents in the ways I imagined one did. As soon as I got back from kayaking, I lay along a bench overlooking the Camel Valley and bought a large pack of non-alcoholic drinks to be delivered home in time for our return. I calculated my due date and signed up to websites, apps and newsletters that offered insights into the likes of my baby's growth, each week comparing the embryo to the size of a different fruit or vegetable. I embraced the consumerist trappings of motherhood with zeal, enjoying daily emails from stores selling irresistible garb with nautical prints and teddy-bear ears.

A stack of new books started to pile up, with titles that appealed to my fondness for planning – *What to Expect When You're Expecting, The Birth of a Mother, Your Baby: Week by Week*. We talked about my maternity leave, planning trips to everywhere from Norfolk to Japan. And I nested, gradually gathering things that looked like the childhood I wanted to provide.

We bought fabric for our baby's bedroom curtains. We hung the sorts of picture we'd had on our own childhood walls – cartoon dogs, naïf cheetahs. We decided to sort out our garden before our hands became too full and while I could still bend over. At the garden centre we bought grasses and herbs, squat pinks and buxom hydrangeas, and – randomly, found alone in an aisle of climbers – a Meyer lemon tree. These fruits, which taste like something in between a lemon and a mandarin, are native to California, a place where a little piece of me will always reside after that year abroad as a student. We planted it in a terracotta pot on our patio. It started to grow in tandem with me.

My pear shape had always given me reason to believe that I was made for baby-making. I have broad hips and thick thighs, and over time I'd come to see myself as breeding stock. There had to be a reason that I was built this way, that I looked so preposterous in a jumpsuit? It had helped me to view aspects of my body I felt less thrilled about through a lens of biological purpose.

But it turned out that I don't love pregnancy and it doesn't feel like a natural condition for me at all. A couple of weeks after Cornwall the nausea starts. No vomiting, luckily, but constant seasickness that only fades with crackers and grapefruit.

For Freddie, the baby is just a concept in those early days of pregnancy. Without morning sickness, it might have been the same for me. Feeling ill is a reminder that I am pregnant because otherwise, life seems to continue as normal. I go to work, look the same, wear all my regular clothes. What I lose in gastric vigour, I gain in not having periods.

At the twelve-week scan, I see Freddie's eyes fill with tears at the sight of the cannellini bean onscreen. The sonographer points out the baby's bulbous head, the quiver of a heartbeat, and its bladder, which, from its dark colour, she can tell is full. She gives us a printout of an ultrasound still. We give our parents a glimpse of their first grandchild and break the news to siblings and friends.

The following day I feel queasier than usual. I stay in bed with a bag of crisps and YouTube, but I start to feel worse. I throw up. It's a really hot summer and I wind up in hospital on a drip for the afternoon. It's a nasty bug. Rehydration fluids and paracetamol sort me out, but the episode heralds a new stage of pregnancy. I order a 'Baby on Board' badge from Transport for London and start to slow down.

I like my second trimester. The sickness subsides at fourteen weeks and I enjoy food again. I am full of energy at work. I indulge my cravings. I pre-emptively buy a sausage-shaped pillow to train myself to sleep on my side. I feel on top of the world – capable, strong, happy.

The twenty-week scan confirms our instinct that we are having a girl. With the graduation from 'it' to 'she', the baby's personhood evolves. I love looking at her stuck to our fridge door, at her undulating profile, retroussé nose, puckered lips. So this is who's been demanding all that grapefruit. We discuss names. There are a handful of options that we both like. We're superstitious about calling her something before she arrives, but there's a standout name that we both love. It's mooted and hovers there for the rest of my pregnancy, practised in my head countless times, tested alongside different middle and surname options in my iPhone Notes.

My body is visibly changing now, although I'm still pretty mobile. We go away for a long weekend and though I look inflated in my swimming costume, my belly pulling the seams into my groin for an excellent double bum, I do wonder if I look six months' pregnant. But I've heard that much of the baby's growth happens in the final trimester. What's more, this is my first baby, and my ab muscles (ancient history at the time of writing) are taut, a resistance band to tiny kicks and the slow forming of life. Worries float into my head and out again, because everything's probably alright, because things usually are. As my pregnancy advances further, I start to have frightening visions of tripping on a tree root when I'm walking the dog, or of dropping my newborn daughter. I tell Freddie and he says he thinks this must be normal – we have a big responsibility ahead of us, it's natural to feel nervous.

I'm not particularly worried about the size of my bump because I feel huge. I graduate to maternity trousers, and I care less and less about how I look. I find this refreshing. Everything I do – getting an Uber home instead of the train at night, eating a bar of chocolate when I crave sugar – feels somehow noble, necessary. I start to get twinges in my sciatic nerve, develop jowls and feel, as they say, 'increased foetal movement'. The baby kicks a lot, often when music is playing, particularly when Freddie plays the guitar next to me.

My work often means we go out in town, so we neglect the local places we might otherwise use more. Our neighbours are nice but at a different life stage and we haven't made any new friends since moving in. Antenatal classes seem like a good idea. We sign up for NCT and, a couple of weeks after Christmas, when I'm thirty or so weeks pregnant, we start meeting with a group of seven other couples expecting their first babies in February and March.

There is something faintly comical about sixteen adults sitting in a circle with a teacher, who has handed each couple a felt-tip pen and a piece of card on which to write their names, their due dates and what kind of baby they are expecting, if they know. I feel like we could be in a sitcom, thrown together in a room with a bunch of couples who happened to have unprotected sex at the same time as us. Except not necessarily, because our group paints a mixed picture of modern parenthood; among us, there's a lesbian couple, another mum is non-binary, another still carrying a baby conceived with a donor egg. Not to mention all the different careers people have, with some, like me, working in the media, but also a few of what, in just over a year, we will all come to refer to as key workers: there's a specialist oncology nurse, a social worker, an occupational therapist. Admittedly, we are, across the board, middle class: NCT classes are not available on the NHS. However, insofar as a group of middle-class millennials can be diverse, ours is.

Antenatal classes are designed to appeal to those who like to prepare and plan – the pillars on which successful careers have been built – even if having a baby is, fundamentally, unplannable. We want a curriculum and we get one. I can't say it isn't fun. There are always biscuits. We learn good trivia, such as how the raised bumps around a woman's nipples are called Montgomery's tubercles; there is a class on nappy changing, which we practise on dolls wearing nappies that our tutor has creatively filled with condiments denoting different digestive symptoms in a newborn. A breastfed baby's poo should look like piccalilli.

My concern about the size of my bump returns in the penultimate NCT meeting. Great heaving stomachs surround me, while mine remains tidily encased in my childbearing hips. Lots of people outside of this room have told me how 'neat' I am, as though it's a compliment; is skinniness the gold standard even in pregnancy, I wonder? Perhaps it's people's way of being nice, given that I'm clearly not, as they say, 'blooming'.

My baby has the last due date of the group, so I reassure myself that she has a little more time to grow than the others. I'm also aware that the position of the foetus has a bearing on how you show, as does, apparently, the sex. You're supposedly less likely to have a poppy-out shelf-like bump if you're expecting a girl, for example.

And, again, I *feel* enormous, increasingly so, hauling arse, thighs and tummy around with me. To my office in King's Cross and back. To Rome on an assignment. I even have a job interview, entirely in denial about the fact that imminent maternity leave probably precludes me taking it if I get it (I don't). I am exhausted but also energised, especially by the baby's movements, to which I have become accustomed. I think I will miss them when she's out. She flits between graceful swirls and assertive thumps, and Freddie and I enjoy the spectacle of her nightly round of hiccups popping on my abdomen.

At our thirty-four-week appointment, my midwife measures my bump. They call this measurement 'fundal height' – from the approximate top of the uterus to the pubic bone – and in the latter stages of pregnancy, they expect it to be as many centimetres as you are weeks pregnant, plus or minus 2 cm. I am measuring about 31 cm, a little small, and the midwife suggests I go for an extra scan, hastening to add that she's not worried. This is for peace of mind, she says. The opportunity to see my daughter (*my daughter!*) onscreen another time is exciting, and the scan is booked for in a few days' time in early February.

The night before the scan, I go to a dinner hosted by one of my columnists, known for hearty, colourful vegetarian food that seduces even the most seasoned of meat eaters. It is a beautiful evening, candlelit, everything gorgeously styled, with a group of dynamic, well-presented women who work in food and publishing. There is palpable excitement for me about becoming a mother, even from those I don't know. It is touching and, when I leave, I feel high. I think this might be the last time that things feel normal.

Freddie comes with me to the scan. The sonographer is not very chatty and spends a long time pressing into my abdomen, stopping to re-gel a couple of times. He and the nurse mutter things I don't understand to one another while we stare at the screen, hoping to glimpse the baby's face. Is that my mouth? I think I can see Freddie's frown! Eventually we are told there's a Doppler reading that's 'a bit high', but that this could be because the baby is constricting the umbilical cord somehow, squeezing it in her little hand, perhaps. They recommend we come back for another scan in a week or two.

Lewisham Hospital sends us away with our orange book containing all my notes from the midwife and ultrasound paperwork, the latest of which shows the sonographer's findings plotted on to graphs. I don't even know what Dopplers are, but when I look it up, I learn that they measure blood flow in various blood vessels. There is one reading, known as PI (pulsatility index), for the baby's umbilical cord, that is very high – above 95 per cent, which looks to be off the chart – higher than the 'bit high' they quoted to me. Google informs me that this reading is often associated with foetal growth restriction but – my tidy bump notwithstanding – this baby has been growing steadily. She's certainly not big, but nor is she teeny.

Freddie and I react to this news in ways true to our separate, fundamental natures – and opposite to each other. These differences are best illustrated by an experience we had early in our relationship. We'd gone to the Lake District for the weekend and, on a walk designed to work up an appetite for dinner, found ourselves on a footpath through a field of young bull calves, who were initially curious, then enraged about us being in their space. Adrenaline flooded my veins, flight instinct took over and I started to run, screaming, 'Fuck! Fuck! Fuck!' as I pulled a sanguine Freddie downhill, the bullocks cantering towards us. Having clambered over the wall, the high drama faded behind me and I was ready for a drink. Only then did the fear catch up with Freddie. He relived how frightened he'd felt for days afterwards. My husband, I learnt, is great in a crisis but suffers afterwards.

So when we are told that we need to be monitored for these last weeks of pregnancy, I feel instantly that familiar heat of high alert, but am quickly reassured by the soothing coos of clinicians. Freddie, meanwhile, leaves the sonography department and frets. We both know his mind now won't rest until the baby arrives.

Another two weeks pass. My mum comes with me to the next scan. I encourage Fred to stay at work because this isn't a major cause for concern – it's *good* they're monitoring me – and I rather like the idea of Mum getting a glimpse of her granddaughter before she arrives. As always when we are alone and passing time together, we do the *Guardian* crossword while we wait to be called in. With life about to become more demanding, every such moment feels precious.

After the scan, we see a doctor who tells me that everything is fine, that the reading has come down enough for her to be happy to discharge me. Whether it was the desire to see the baby onscreen one last time, or the flicker of something else which prompts me to ask for another scan, I can't say. But I request one and they are happy to oblige an anxious almost-mother.

Freddie comes this time. I can tell I'm getting used to this place, as the hospital's confusing corridor system now feels quite familiar. The ultrasound shows that the Doppler is very high again and we are told to go up to the maternity unit to see a doctor. We have a long wait and eat supper from a vending machine. I wish I'd made sandwiches.

Eventually a young obstetrician calls us over to a bed and draws the curtain around us. The baby has gone into 'brain-saving mode', she tells us, and the advice is to induce me tomorrow, Saturday, when my pregnancy hits term at thirty-seven weeks. Come in at 9 p.m., she says, and we'll get going.

Several years later, I will speak to Dr Spyros Bakalis, a foetal medicine doctor at St Thomas' Hospital, who levels with me about the limitations of what can be known about a baby before it is born. Short of invasive prenatal testing like amniocentesis, they have only ultrasound, which looks at anatomy and blood flow to assess a foetus's wellbeing. 'There's not much else we can do,' he tells me, meaning that if there's a whiff of something awry, they 'shoot first and ask questions later'. In cases like ours, where something is not right but it's not obvious what, close monitoring and, if necessary, early delivery are the only options.

In the next twenty-four hours, our last at home as a couple without children, I hand over at work, and we pack bags and make arrangements for the dog. I hadn't imagined being induced, hadn't even read up on what it involves, I'd just assumed that my birth plan would come good. I don't feel upset, though. 'Brain-saving' sounds ominous but the doctor had delivered the information calmly. It doesn't necessarily mean that anything is wrong, she told me, just that all placentas have a lifespan, and mine might have reached its own. Every parent I've spoken to has had some sort of drama around delivery. This is ours. If anything, I feel lucky – lucky that the hospital can move quickly, and that we'll be meeting our daughter three weeks earlier than expected.

Everything and nothing happens in the next three days. Attempts at induction fail to get labour going. Two pessaries, a gel, lots of poking around. Neither the baby nor I are ready for a rude awakening, it would seem.

The plan I'd made with my midwife was for a vaginal birth in the midwife-led hospital birth centre, which in the pictures looked a bit like a decent, if slightly kinky, hotel room, with its red spotlights and water tub. Up on the labour ward, however, the things we had prepared are off limits. I understand the reasons for this – my preferred conditions for birth may be different from other people's – but I'm disappointed not to hear Freddie's 'Good Contractions' playlist or burn clary sage like the earth mother I like to think I am.

Despite being told to come in at 9 p.m., my induction isn't started until 3 a.m., and meds are then administered every twenty-four hours, so our hospital experience becomes quite nocturnal and we are tired before there's even been a contraction. Freddie sleeps beside me on a yoga mat for the first couple of nights, but goes home for the third, returning with a tub of curry the next day. After several days of hospital meals, this feels like the most romantic thing he has ever done.

I am largely alright because I'm the patient. Watching Freddie, I can see how hard it is to be the partner, without a bed or catering, with such a vested interest but so little say. We are both keen for the baby to arrive and for the three of us to get home. My body, however, just doesn't respond to the induction meds. By Wednesday, a caesarean is strongly recommended and after some deliberation, and gentle encouragement from my mum over WhatsApp, we accept it.

Freddie puts on scrubs and chats to one anaesthetist while the other talks me through what's going to happen. He gives me an epidural and spritzes me with cold spray until I cannot feel anything. There is the humming of ambient machinery and the stark reflection of halogen light on steel surfaces. The process seems impossibly calm – smooth, even – in comparison with the Hollywood-style vaginal birth I'd anticipated. Behind a screen of scrub fabric, there's some tugging, some rooting, and then a sudden squawk.

Love set you going like a fat gold watch, wrote Sylvia Plath.

Suddenly, there's another person in the room.

'So . . . is she? Shall we?' asks Freddie.

I nod, unable to take my eyes off our baby lying beside us in a Perspex cot. She is still coiled up, hands together in front of her like a squirrel taking pause. 'I think so,' I whisper.

'Hello, Vida,' we both say, softly.

She has a lot of very dark hair. Her nose is an acorn, her lips turn down just like Freddie's when he's asleep, her heavy, soft eyelids open to reveal grey-green irises. Imagine, I think, never to have seen before. Or to have heard anything except pulse and womb sounds, voices muffled by layers of muscle and skin. How uncomplicated, too, to have such clear priorities: air, food, sleep. In the recovery room, after I have been sewn up, her mouth roots around then latches on to me hungrily. Gently but confidently, she takes her first gulps of colostrum before falling back to sleep in my arms, nestling in the institutional blankets.

I had spent eight months wondering what our child would look like, unable to picture the cross of Freddie and me, but now that she is here, it seems so inevitable, so obvious. I can't imagine her looking any other way. And already, she is so much herself.

We have been given a private room and our parents and my brother come briefly with hummus and loud voices before being chucked out by a disapproving midwife. I enjoy these hours, shell-shocked yet high on morphine and relief.

Freddie, the baby and I settle down for a sleepless yet strangely peaceful night. She is sleepy but doesn't like to be put down for long. This is fine with us, and we take it in turns to practise cradling her, engaging new muscles. We whisper her name a lot, repetition binding the word to her form. By morning, she is Vida.

A foetus is a tiny burglar, a parasite of sorts, its mother quite literally its lifeblood while she is pregnant. A transaction happens in the placenta, an exchange of blood: the mother's is rich in oxygen, while the baby's is expert at binding itself to that oxygen, thanks to haemoglobin F, a foetal form of haemoglobin, the blood protein which transports oxygen around the body. For this reason, women need to produce significantly more blood during pregnancy. The needs of the foetus will always be prioritised over hers – the maternal sacrifice starts early! – and so she often becomes anaemic.

I wasn't surprised, then, to learn that I was anaemic after Vida's birth; my midwife had prepared me for the possibility.

What's more, throughout my adult life, my iron levels had been on the low side; it made sense that pregnancy had eaten into my reserves and left me lacking.

The doctor came in to tell me I would need to take iron supplements – an easy fix. Anaemia leaves you feeling tired, and I definitely felt that. I lay in a hospital bed, hooked up to a catheter, and was brought water and snacks on demand while my baby – my own micro-parasite – slept or fed on me. You can rob me of oxygen any time you like, I think, breathing in her sweetness. Thank goodness you're here – and that you're OK.

The peace of Vida's first night is short-lived. Six days in hospital have caught up with Freddie and me, and we are itching to get home. An SHO (a senior house officer, a level of junior doctor) wearing red tights does Vida's newborn check and tells us that she has a heart murmur. Either this is something normal and common, she says, and will right itself over the coming weeks, or it could be a very rare condition, which could be further indicated by testing the discrepancy between the pulses in her legs and arms. Perhaps it's my state of mind, but it all seems garbled and unclear. My baby is perfect – look at her! I'm confident that the SHO is just being overzealous, university lectures still fresh in her memory.

We go up to the neonatal intensive care unit for Vida to have her pulses taken, yet another complication to what we'd assumed would be a straightforward birth. Vida is placed in another Perspex cot while a nurse tries to get readings from her tiny blood vessels as she writhes around in protest. She has been prised from the womb before she was ready, cutting short valuable fattening-up time; not only has she had to meet her parents three weeks early, not only must she learn to breathe and eat, she's now being prodded by strangers. She opens her mouth and emits a creak of objection. I tell myself that she won't remember this and the doctors and nurses must do whatever is necessary. I hold Freddie's hand as his eyes fill with tears; we look at Vida, swimming in a newborn-sized sleepsuit, neon orange with black cats on it. We'll be home soon, I remind him.

But not that soon. We have to stay another night and have another assessment tomorrow. The same SHO tells me she isn't happy with how infrequently Vida has been feeding, so now I must make sure she breastfeeds every two hours.

Freddie goes home for some sleep and I stay in hospital to do the opposite, because Vida's second night in the world is very different from her first. Turns out twenty-four hours can change everything: she is only happy to sleep in my arms, her body buoyed by the undulations of my breath, soothed by the white noise of my body, now experienced from the outside. And the two-hour feeding regimen is punishing.

I try putting her down, allowing her to suck on my little finger in lieu of a nipple, gradually withdrawing it to fresh cries. At about 4 a.m., I pick up my phone and buy a dummy online. I hadn't imagined using one, but I hadn't wanted a caesarean either. Yet here we are. Clearly, I have learnt the lesson of doing whatever I need to do to stay alive/sane/well pretty quickly.

The next day my mum comes to spend the morning with us armed, as ever, with a crossword and a loaf of banana bread. The day outside is piercingly bright and I take some pictures of Mum by a window, Vida slumped over her shoulder like a miniature sloth. We wrap her in a blanket Mum had used when I was a baby, and she cradles her in the corner of the room for an hour while I try to sleep.

I drift into a doze, only to be roused by a small choir outside the room singing 'Let's Go Fly a Kite' from *Mary Poppins*. The combination of the song, nostalgically euphoric, with the choir's harmonies and the presence of my baby is almost unbearable. My heart soars with the lyrics.

Freddie comes back, marginally better rested but the wind still out of his sails. He makes it known to the SHO (today in mustard tights) just how much we want to go home. This is all too much, he says. We are confused by the cocktail of messages we're hearing from doctors: some reassuring, others diligently acting on their concerns. Eventually we are summoned for another round of pulse checks – and the discrepancy between arms and legs is less alarming. Finally we can leave.

There's no getting around Vida's heart murmur, however. It will most likely resolve itself, they say, but we will be asked back in six weeks to have a check-up: they'll send us a letter. Seven days, six nights, five midwives, four curries, three cannulas, two pessaries and one caesarean later, we go home with our baby.

My mother-in-law, Louise, opens our front door and the smell of roast chicken wafts out. Ernie trots over, tail wagging frantically after our week apart, nose sniffing curiously at the bundle that Freddie carries in. I've wanted this moment so desperately. Let's go fly a kite.

I spend hours chanting lullabies to Vida. Breathlessly, because I'm almost always bouncing up and down on an inflated rubber birthing ball, hoping that the motion will soothe her cries.

It's eleven weeks in and there's none of the serenity with which she arrived. My dad loves to say that there's nothing wrong with her lungs, which in spite of the subtext – that his first grandchild makes a shit ton of noise that we can't seem to stop – I find strangely comforting, as though her near-constant crying is indicative of good health and spirit.

Doubt tugs at me, though. She often screams, writhes, creases up her face and bawls. Most of all when we coax her to feed. These days, most of our afternoons are like this, maybe with a short nap in my armpit after a harrowing session of trying to get my boob into her mouth. We have mixed success with this, but she seems less and less inclined to do it. When she does feed, it doesn't last long.

I use these moments to escape – into *Fleabag*, perhaps, which nudges me to find some kind of hilarity in the darkness I feel, or Netflix's *Selling Sunset*, all cat fights and hair extensions, which suddenly makes the sight of my baby, her perfect form clad only in natural fibres, calming. Until she wakes and starts to cry again.

At night, after she's been bathed and dressed, it takes at least half an hour of bouncing and chanting alongside the white noise of a blasting hairdryer to get her to latch. I console myself with tenuous positives. Maybe I'll reclaim some core strength! Sometimes I even repeat to myself the words proffered by Lactation Lydia – a nickname which stuck for the kindly Lewisham breastfeeding consultant who squirted out reassurance – that Vida is probably just a very efficient feeder. She'll be getting what she needs!

But surely she's hungry? Irrespective of how I would feel about a giant, weeping nipple being shoved in my face, isn't she supposed to want this? But she screams. And screams. Should I take it personally? Does my milk taste bad? How ironic, to have a mother who prides herself on her cooking but can't make good milk.

When she does, finally, latch on, I set the stopwatch on my phone. Anything north of five minutes satisfies me; seven is really good, I think, with Lactation Lydia's advice front of mind. When the NCT WhatsApp chat pings with notes about the likes of hour-long bedtime feeds, I try to disregard the flutter of worry.

Four minutes, thirty-six seconds. I feel Vida's wet mouth loosen around me: she's gone to sleep. A few sucks and sheer exhaustion have finally knocked her out. I put her down in her cot and creep out of the room, the precise points at which every floorboard creaks now written into my sensory memory.

The night shift has begun. I have a moment's peace before the charade starts all over again in the small hours of fairy lights and gobbled-down granola (because even when your baby won't feed, breastfeeding is hungry work).

Freddie's return to work was tough. Because he runs his own business, he had been able to take a month off, and before Vida was born, I'd felt confident that I would have got the hang of things in those four weeks. But I hadn't, and in the final few days of his paternity leave, I was acutely aware that time was running out. We were so far from having established a feeding routine that I hadn't dared to leave the house alone. Plus I had no mode of transport: I was scared of dropping her when I put the sling on, and she screamed blue murder in the bassinet of the pram. Freddie, it seemed to me, was going to work for a rest, and I'm sure the reality of going to his studio to make music for eight hours a day did offer an escape. But it was bittersweet – he was exhausted and, increasingly, worried about my fragility. Before this, I don't think he'd ever have described me as 'fragile'.

I was just about managing to meet Vida's basic needs – changing her nappies, feeding her for as long as she would, allowing her to sleep on me – but ignoring my own. Before she was born, we'd bought a rocker so that I might be able to put her down while I made lunch, went to the loo, let the dog out, but once Freddie was back at work, cooking was unthinkable, and Ernie and I spent much of those weeks with our legs crossed until we were relieved by one of my parents. I could only summon them over so much, though. I knew my mum could see I was finding it hard, had spotted my flickers of panic when Vida wouldn't stay latched. She always came with soup and can-do spirit, but also a belief, I sensed, that I was gradually adapting to one of the biggest transitions of adult life. Her presence was usually restorative, and I encouraged her to go home after tea, only to feel totally at sea again as soon as she did.

According to the books and my NCT friends, five o'clock is a baby's 'witching hour'. I couldn't see much difference between 5 p.m. and the rest of the day. It was still another hour until Freddie got home and it was a desperate one. I would try feeding and Vida would roar at the suggestion of my boobs. I'd open a book – *Guess How Much I Love You?* – and try to lull her with talk of nut-brown hares in my best ASMR voice. She bellowed throughout and I gave up. Ernie often stood next to the sofa and met my gaze, his eyes forlorn. Once I was sure I saw him shake his head.

When Freddie arrived home, the crying became a problem shared. He'd put something in the oven and between us we would wash, feed and cradle Vida to sleep for a few hours. Despite the might of her lungs, she was still tiny, tiny enough to kip next to us in the SleepyHead pod on the sofa until we went to bed. Everything instantly felt so much better when Freddie was there that I started to dread his departure the next day as soon as he walked through the door. Just as I have acquired a dependant, I have become one myself, I thought.

—

Gradually, the other women in my NCT group are getting the hang of things. Routines begin to emerge as they learn to pre-empt their babies' appetites and sleeping patterns.

Some of them are using apps – Little Ones, Baby Buddy; others swear by controversial child-sleep expert Gina Ford; others still follow no particular doctrine except the belief that they and their babies will find their way.

All the above are yet to work for me. With every failed new tack comes a fresh wave of defeat. I'm no good at this. I like to be good at things. I have been known to leave a tennis court with a smashed racket. But I can't leave this court. Every day, multiple times, I confront my maternal failures.

Freddie stokes the fortune of Jeff Bezos and invests in a gamut of accoutrements for baby sleep hygiene and colic-friendly feeding. Swaddles and gripe water; dummies and Ewan the Sheep, a white-noise toy; virtually every brand of bottle on the market and a strapless bra for milk expressing, out of which my areoles peep in a way that might, in another universe, be erotic – or funny, at least.

But the baby won't nap. The baby won't feed. The baby is miserable.

Yet, between crying fits, she manages smiles. We have photos as proof: there she is, tracing-paper white but beaming in her floral bloomers. The camera tells lies, though. And we told lies to ourselves.

I look at those pictures now and am haunted by Vida's ghost-like form. Her pallor is unmissable to my now-trained eyes.

But then it was, arguably, easy to miss. Freddie and I saw her every day, her grandparents only a little less often, and its onset was slow.

Much about how we appeared in those early weeks would have seemed normal to the healthcare professionals we saw: a wobbly 'Mum' (because that's always who you are, despite your name being right there on their notes in front of them), easily given to tears; an agitated 'Dad', heavy with new responsibility; a 'fussy' baby that shook its head and cried at the suggestion of feeding.

It was standard stuff. What's more, we were complimented on Vida's beauty, her porcelain skin, her enthusiasm for feeding when she had just been born, and her 'really hydrated' blood when the midwife pricked her heel at just a few days old, to test for – irony of ironies – some (but not all) blood disorders.

As far as I knew, having a baby just *was* this hard. So I lapped up all the positive feedback I could find, believed that this was to be expected, that things would change soon.

If you're in the unusual situation of having a baby that's in a gradual state of decline, you have none of the drama of a stomach bug or a terrible accident, just a draining away of vitality. That something was gravely wrong was not obvious, but its possibility did hang around me like one of the many bad smells that circulated in those first months of breastfeeding – milky muslins, milky nappies, my own milk-soaked nightwear. 'Mother's intuition', you might say, but how does quiet intuition stand a chance amid the din of reassurance and denial?

Postnatal services are largely run by experienced people who are not doctors. Like Lactation Lydia, they ooze motivational comfort to dizzy new parents. And a boost of confidence from someone who knows their stuff is not to be undervalued; the positive things I was told about Vida's progress at that time stuck with me. 'Look at those rubber-band wrists!' 'That's a good, firm latch!' 'It looks like she might have some mild tongue-tie – let's get that sorted.'

Often, wise words like these are all harried mums need to hear, helping you convert crippling anxiety into a normal part of your story, which you'll swap with other mothers over wine in the months to come.

Lactation Lydia refers us to the tongue-tie clinic at King's College Hospital in south-east London. Tongue tie is a condition in which the tongue is tethered to the bottom of the mouth by a short, thick or tight frenulum. It can debilitate a baby's ability to feed and is distressing for mother and baby alike. It's also easy to fix – with a frenotomy, the cutting of the frenulum to release the tongue – so the baby can suck to its heart, mouth and stomach's delight. I see several mothers emerge from the consulting room that day, their baby's feeding transformed.

Obviously, we hope that Vida is tongue-tied, a problem easily solved.

But our appointment is inconclusive and we leave without the procedure. Why make her cry more?

And the problem that is so hard to put a finger on, or put a name to, continues. For now, the tongue-tie is my own.

We spend more and more time at Freddie's mum Louise's house in north London. Hands are a valuable currency these days and an extra pair is priceless. She lives close to his studio, which means I gain two hours more of Freddie a day, and I see Louise for ten minutes every hour, in between her psychotherapy patients – little base-touches of soup, tea and companionship that make me realise how isolated I'd been at our flat.

Though I haven't weighed her in a few weeks, I am almost certain Vida's weight has plateaued. I take her to a children's centre off Abbey Road, hoping it will put my mind at rest. She refuses a feed before we leave, then screams, strapped to me, all the way there. My chest is so tight – it's just the sling, I tell myself. It's like a corset.

Another mum is ahead of us in the weighing queue. Afterwards, she does her baby back up into an oatmeal-coloured onesie, then tucks him into a tie-up sling (mummy bloggers make this look easy – it isn't) and throws an oversized parka over her lithe frame. *Childbearing, moi?* The baby is wide-eyed and smiling adorably.

Our turn comes and I'm right: no weight gain. I express my worries about Vida's weight to the benevolent woman doing the weighing, all dangly earrings and community spirit. She asks me to come outside with her, then heaves a sigh of relief. In the sports-hall glare, she says, my baby was a bit yellow, but in daylight she looks fine.

Mr Sun, Sun, Mr Golden Sun
Please shine down on me

We are back in south London and my friend Sophie is leading a baby massage class for the NCT group. It's a room of fast-fattening babies – they range from six to twelve weeks – and mums who are finding themselves again, gracefully emerging from the 'fourth trimester' in lipstick and with artfully tousled hair.

Mr Sun, Sun, Mr Golden Sun
Hiding behind a tree

I watch, incredulous, as one baby necks 240 ml of formula milk. Another's cries are soothed simply by the expulsion of a heavy load, to which her mother dutifully attends. Another still, wearing a mini tracksuit that mirrors his mum's, happily scoffs at her chest and so misses most of the class, while the other babies wriggle with delight, coo, enjoy the dulcet tones of Sophie's voice.

These little babies are asking you
To please come out so they can play with you

Vida doesn't. I simply cannot stop her crying.

We leave the room and she cries outside for the rest of the class. Afterwards, we all go for a coffee and she thrashes so much that I spill mine.

Her six-week check at the GP happens to have been booked for just after baby massage, so I make my excuses and leave. Vida wails all the way there.

Mr Sun, Sun, Mr Golden Sun
Please shine down on me.

The six-week check – which actually happens at nine weeks, six weeks from my due date rather than from Vida's birth date, for reasons that are unclear – is uneventful. Sophie, Vida's godmother, has come with, and takes pictures of the baby on my lap throughout. When I look at them now, Vida looks a kind of light grey, even in the April sunlight streaming through the doctor's window, her grey-green eyes and dark hair in high contrast to pale, pale skin.

'How's it going?' asks the GP (a trainee, I later learn).

'Well,' I say, 'getting easier.' This is how we now automatically respond to any such question. Why wasn't I honest? We wanted to believe it. And we *did* believe things were getting easier. I spoke with a thicker skin, and lips hardened to the chap of sleep deprivation, ears acclimatised to my baby's persistent cries.

I mention the heart. The GP has a listen and, while she can hear it, she reassures me that it's pretty normal at Vida's age. I want to linger for more encouragement but feel like she's keen to see her next patient.

Sophie comes home with us and stays for bath and bedtime. What kind of an advertisement am I for motherhood? Cow-heavy, as Sylvia Plath described the new mother in 'Morning Song', breast hanging out of my nursing garb, which I shakily steer into the baby's mouth. My friend sees my elaborate evening routine, the hair dryer, the rain app, Ewan the bloody sheep, the bouncing, the bouncing, the interminable bouncing. Only later, once her goddaughter had been diagnosed, did the horror of that afternoon make sense to her.

We go back to Lewisham Hospital to have Vida's heart murmur checked. A routine appointment.

First things first, I strip her down, place her on the scales. This time, she's lost weight.

The paediatrician gingerly listens to Vida's chest, peels her bottom eyelashes back to reveal the membranes of her lower lids. She looks at her, hands her back to me.

'Sit down, please,' she says.

She wanders round to the desk opposite our chairs, pulls her knees underneath it, clears her throat, 'OK, so how do *you* think she is doing?'

Her tone digs a moat of fear around me.

'Yeah, good ...' stutters Freddie, '... things are getting easier ...'

The doctor interrupts. 'She is *very pale. VERY an-ae-mic. Did you not see?*'

The wall, the ceiling, faces and furniture begin to melt.

'This baby has to be admitted now,' she says. 'She needs a blood transfusion urgently.'

And in that instant, the world changes forever.

After

Paediatric inpatients. From here, I look back on our anxious days in the maternity unit almost nostalgically. Cheery midwives have become serious doctors who don't yet have answers; battered wipe-clean toys replace brand new baby kit; and I am no longer the patient with the cannula – my daughter is.

The consultant had been quick to tell us that Vida needed a blood transfusion urgently, but the route to this happening is unclear. Some of her blood is drawn, the first of many attempts at wrangling her small veins, which are unforthcoming with their contents. It seems absurd to be removing blood from a body which, by all accounts, doesn't have enough of it.

It is a long day of sitting, pacing, sitting some more. Since our consultation, we have occupied a row of chairs in a corridor, waiting for Vida's blood-test results to formalise the next steps. I am stricken, so tired but unable to keep still. My mum joins us; this time she has brought sandwiches, but we leave the crossword untouched.

At last the consultant finds us to deliver the news: Vida's haemoglobin level, her 'HB', is 29. This means nothing to us, but the doctor grimaces as she explains that it is 'very low', keeping her mouth in an 'O' shape for emphasis after saying it. I am rattled by her expression, but not by the diagnosis of anaemia. I tell Freddie matter-of-factly that I was anaemic as a teenager, which Mum corroborates, and he knows I have been taking iron since my caesarean. Surely we can easily resolve Vida's anaemia with iron supplements? And couldn't I eat more iron-rich foods myself, to improve my milk?

'This isn't going to be about iron,' the consultant meets my eyes again, shakes her head slowly.

She explains that normal haemoglobin levels should sit between 115 and 140, that anything below this is considered anaemic, that generally a level in the 80s needs urgent attention.

29.

Words like 'severe' and 'profound' are used.

'Didn't you see she was pale?' the consultant asks. I recall thinking that my hands looked red next to Vida's body in the bath and putting it down to ageing skin.

She makes no secret of her concern. We come to understand that we have an emergency on our hands. Then she tells us we have to join the queue in paediatric A & E. A queue? In this kind of an emergency? A tiny baby without enough blood? *My* tiny baby?

I am struggling to reconcile the consultant's tone of voice with a long queue of runny noses and bumped heads. Freddie goes down to scope out the waiting time and he's told the wait will be several hours. 'Several hours!' I squeak. Is it not ludicrous for us to wait hours under the circumstances? Surely every minute counts? The consultant seems torn between palpable worry and adherence to process.

She discovers that a registrar whom she knows is on duty in paediatric A & E that day and makes a call, proceeding to explain our situation over the phone in booming whispers. I can't tell if she wants us to hear or not. Mum, who (unlike me) did a proper journalistic training in the seventies, sits with a notepad in one hand, pencil poised in the other. She scribbles in shorthand I can't read. Fred and I take it in turns to hold our girl, whose pallor now seems so obvious.

'But, the bone marrow, the bone marrow . . .' the consultant frets. There is something about her tone, also the image of my granny's dogs gnawing at bones, their tongues intermittently caressing the dark, spongy stuff inside – 'the bone marrow', I hear Granny's voice say – that makes my own blood run cold.

The registrar contact comes good and we are granted a queue jump. This is what we want but it gives me a sinking feeling – Vida is an emergency even by the standards of A & E. We are shuffled into a curtained bay, surrounded by the beeps and clatters of toys, rustling crisp packets, bored wails and – the icing on the proverbial – an actual cake being presented to someone.

It is a nightmarish, halogen-lit hour played out to the tune of 'Happy Birthday'. Cannulating a tiny baby is a difficult task requiring, in Vida's case, four clinicians, two parents and one grandparent. There's the registrar who fast-tracked us in, the SHO who'd done our newborn check all those weeks ago (still in colourful tights), and two nurses. One of the nurses squeezes glucose syrup into Vida's mouth, momentarily distracting her from the 'sharp scratch' of the needle.

Babyhood is undignified at the best of times, but the sight of my own baby, squirming like an upside-down beetle on the couch just before a life-saving blood transfusion – because, clearly, that is what this one will be – is unbearable. She is surrounded by the team, who do their best to get the line in at various different 'sites' – elbows, feet, hands. I'm amazed at how they are able to observe an emergency so coolly, discussing their weekends with simultaneous focus on the job. Freddie is flushed, his cheeks almost mockingly pink next to our daughter. My mum is quiet, refraining from her usual small talk to put people at ease. In a whisper, I ask if this could be leukaemia; they say they think not. While we inhabit this new extreme – parenthood in a different dimension, exposed, beyond rescue, even by our parents or each other – the medics chat away. I imagine it's a way of managing the suffering they see every day.

I stroke Vida's hair, unable to pick her up while they aim for veins. I hope that my proximity, my smell perhaps, is somehow comforting; hers is to me – I breathe in the cereal-milk scent of her head, one of just a few sweetnesses to the last eleven weeks and five days.

'I've never seen a baby with haemoglobin this low,' says the SHO. Sometimes you need someone to talk straight, not least at a time like this, when it seems no one will commit to a theory of what's going on. But the remark shatters something in me, my brittle belief, perhaps, that everything will be alright.

Vida is wearing a beige-and-yellow striped body and leggings, a matching set that I'd bought after poring over options online. Because of the cannula, this is the outfit that she will wear for the whole week that we are here in hospital, and which I will later have no difficulty throwing away. Right now, at her palest, her skin and the outfit's colour scheme are like a neutrals Pantone chart, bereft of pinks and reds. Against both, her hair is goth-dark, her eyes dewy black marbles, her contours hollow. I realise I have been watching the colour drain from her for weeks.

Eventually they get the cannula into her hand and bandage it up into a boxing glove, a fitting costume for a person who, I'm starting to suspect, has spent her whole life fighting.

Vida is admitted to paediatric inpatients and has a blood transfusion in four parts over as many days. They explain that this is because there is only so much blood you can give in one go; that they mustn't overwhelm her little heart with too much fluid, so it must be given very slowly. After just one instalment, she is transformed into a baby that feeds. She latches on with gusto. She sucks and sucks, no dropping off after four minutes. The girl is on a milk marathon.

On the second day, we see some colour in her cheeks, which flush after another feed.

On the third day, her twelve-week birthday, she smiles. Photo evidence even reveals the hint of a chubby cheek. In it, she has the expression of someone in the calm after a storm, which I find both gratifying and troubling. She has been through so much.

On the fourth day, the smiles widen when we sing to her. She loves 'Old MacDonald', my realistic 'woof' and Freddie's deep bass 'oink'. We have also taken to singing Prince's 'The Most Beautiful Girl in the World' to her in the highest pitch we can muster. When we had found out we were expecting a girl, we discussed not praising her for her looks. But it feels important to tell her now, on day five of the striped beige outfit and boxing glove, when Monday's failed attempts at cannulation have started to become little bruises. She is so beautiful. I am reminded of a line in a book by Richard Brautigan; the female protagonist – who shares her name with Vida, no less! – is 'so beautiful that the advertising people would have made her into a national park'. A little objectifying, perhaps, but I'd always liked the sentiment.

The panic we felt on day one quickly gives way to steeliness: we are in the right place and the doctors here will sort this out. I treat it as the mini-break I wouldn't have chosen: we have round-the-clock help and even manage to watch something on BBC iPlayer together (Louis Theroux's film on postpartum psychosis, for a little light viewing). Technically, two parents are not allowed to stay the night with a child here, but they turn a blind eye to Freddie and me sleeping top to toe on the single camp bed next to Vida's cot. I'm grateful for this. Despite having to shape-shift around my husband's knees, I get the best rest I've had in twelve weeks. Vida wakes for one woozy feed in the night, then goes back down. She is peaceful in a way I've not known her – she sleeps, she feeds, she smiles. All this normal baby routine stuff is a revelation.

But the daytimes are something else. It is mid-May: the sun is bright and our room is hot. The windows don't open and there's no air conditioning. Lewisham Hospital had survived plans for the demolition of two-thirds of its buildings a few years ago. It is now in urgent need of funding and attention. Paediatric inpatients overlooks a car park and the bins; I feel trapped in the bowels of the hospital. I long to give Vida a bath and have one myself.

The outside world carries on as usual. On the ward, I procrastinate in my usual ways, online shopping and chipping in to an NCT conversation on WhatsApp, this time about natural baby products. I tap away, explaining self-assuredly why I choose to use a particular nappy cream. I can talk about purchase decisions confidently – nap schedules and feeding routines less so. In the first weeks, there'd been much chat between us all during the small hours, but more recently, other people's babies have been sleeping a little longer. Things seeming to ease for the others made me hope that they would for us soon too, even if they had in fact been getting harder. Now I know something about why.

Vida has a lot of blood tests. The paediatricians explain to us that anaemia can be caused by one of three things: blood loss; the destruction of red blood cells; or decreased or faulty red blood cell production. Understanding what has caused Vida's will be a process of elimination.

They list all the things they are looking for that might explain it, including a common viral illness called parvovirus, which I might have contracted when pregnant and which commonly stops young red cells maturing in the bone marrow for a period of time. There is also the chance that Vida's blood group is incompatible with mine, or that she has internal bleeding. They test both Vida and me for HIV. They make a 'blood film' to look at the cellular composition and anatomy of her blood – among other things, this checks for signs of leukaemia. They of course test her iron levels. There are any number of other procedures, too, ultrasounds to check for blood loss from her liver, kidneys, stomach; an echocardiogram to get a full picture of her heart function, which involves countless wires on sticky pads. For weeks afterwards, I will be picking off residual adhesive from her chest.

Results start trickling in and are either negative or normal. At first, I don't understand why they don't seem more optimistic about this, feeling only immense relief that they are confident that Vida doesn't have blood cancer. But as more and more reasons for such severe anaemia are ruled out, I start to feel uneasy. I sense there's another possibility lurking in the shadows. The consultant's conversation with the registrar a few days ago comes back to me. *The bone marrow.*

At one point I am looking over some of Vida's notes, including the results of her newborn check. In them, the SHO describes her as 'pink', one sign of a healthy baby. I also notice that her haemoglobin at birth was 115. I hadn't realised they'd even tested this at the time, and I start to research the normal HB range for a newborn baby. As I now know, by both adult and paediatric standards, 115 isn't alarmingly low, but in neonates it seems to be very much under the expected level. I ask about this, why hadn't it been flagged up at the time? I'm told it wouldn't have been deemed low enough to cause alarm.

Both Freddie's mother and mine are keen for us to be transferred to Great Ormond Street, for Vida to be at a specialist children's hospital. We need a paediatric haematologist. Trouble is, Lewisham doesn't have one. Our only access to blood expertise is via a very busy adult haematologist who is conferring with the Evelina, the children's hospital at St Thomas' in Lambeth. We suggest that they refer us directly to the Evelina, given Vida is currently confounding the doctors here. The long chain of communication also seems to be prolonging the uncertainty, but Freddie and I are anxious about making the team who have looked after us feel undermined.

I make a point of offering snacks to the doctors when they come in. I ask the SHO where she lives, drop little details about myself into conversation, show her a photo of Ernie. We're about the same age. I was friends with some medics at uni. In another context, we might have crossed paths. I want her to see me, to know who I am outside of this hospital. Maybe if I assert that version of myself enough, maybe this one – the hollow mother of the baby with the lowest haemoglobin she's ever seen – will go away.

The transfusions have brought Vida's HB back into the normal range (just), and Lewisham agree that we may leave, on the understanding that we return for blood tests twice a week for the foreseeable. She's got enough blood; now we have to see what she does with it. It's a watch-and-wait situation.

We pack our bags and Vida's boxing glove is unwound into a pile of lint bandage. A teddy-bear sticker holding the cannula in position is peeled back and the line removed. Her hand is very bruised. We can finally change her clothes and put her liberated right arm through the sleeve of a babygrow. While we wait for formal confirmation of our discharge, I take her on a walk around the ward to look at the murals of cartoon characters.

We are handed a discharge summary, which I shove into Vida's red book of growth charts and immunisation records. We hurry out to the car and, for the second time in three months, go home with our daughter, feeling huge relief.

I can't say it feels the same as the first time, though.

It's a beautiful spring and our garden is starting to bloom. Bees spiral around untamed herbs, and the Meyer lemon's tough green fruits continue to expand. Louise is staying with us, and on the Friday she welcomes us back with her vegetarian shepherd's pie. My mum pops round the next day with French onion soup and a polenta cake. All these are signature comfort foods, which silently remind us that Vida is not the only child here. Between us there is the understanding that language will return when things are clearer. For now, we have food.

I am relieved to be home, but what we gain in comfort, we lose in institutional support. Much as we had wanted to be discharged, the hospital had offered us a framework. Here there are no doctors around to field my questions, no nurses popping in for regular 'sets of obs' (to take Vida's temperature, blood pressure and oxygen saturation). I realise that now it is up to us to assess the situation for ourselves, to watch our baby for pallor, fast breathing, irritability, and to sound the alarm if we are worried. But we hadn't spotted it before – how could I be sure that we wouldn't miss something again? *Didn't you see she was pale?*

On the Saturday, Louise goes to a friend's wedding in Suffolk, promising to come back the next day. She leaves us drinking coffee with my mum. I regularly steal away to the loo to consult my phone, typing in Vida's symptoms, also 'high umbilical PI Doppler', feeling a hunch that her anaemia must in some way be linked to those funny scans that prompted the earlier-than-planned delivery. My reading makes Freddie nervous; he fears, I think, the places it might take me – or indeed where it might take us, should I unearth something. Mum is better versed in my tendency toward self-diagnosis, gently prising my phone away when she catches me in the act.

I see Vida's red book with the hospital paperwork tucked inside it on the living-room table, untouched since our return yesterday. I pick it up and pull out the discharge summary in case it has more clues which might inform internet searches. There, in black and white, are the facts: my daughter's name, her date of birth, her NHS number. Among the data and acronyms, a word stands out. *Palliative.*

Technically, the word is not written in bold, but its assembly of letters has that effect, jumping off the page assertively.

I scan the page again.

I hadn't seen it wrong; my eyes zoom in on it.

Palliative, it says. Right next to 'Specialism at Discharge'. It states that Vida is now under the palliative care team. Palliative care, making the incurable comfortable. Palliative, an adjective reserved for neither life nor death, but a kind of purgatory; a purgatory experienced by the critically, complicatedly ill.

Had Vida been diagnosed with something that we hadn't been told about? As far as I knew, this was the first time this word had been used.

It's a Saturday, meaning the ward will be virtually unreachable by phone. Still, I try, hoping for answers, and can't get through. Terror fizzes in my stomach, reacting chemically with the exhaustion of five days in hospital.

'Surely it's a mistake,' Mum says.

'Let's deal with what's in front of us,' says Fred, a favourite saying of his mum's, which will become like a mantra to us in the coming weeks. He means we mustn't draw conclusions until we've spoken to Lewisham. I realise that's unlikely to happen for another two days and I wonder how I will survive the uncertainty for so long.

Louise returns from the wedding, energised by twenty-four hours of distraction. She is full of stories – of outfits and eccentric old classmates not seen for forty years. Normally I'd feast on these details, but I can't really listen. I sit and twitch. My eye sockets feel hollow; I can't catch my breath; I am only really conscious of the fizzing.

Louise has since described what she saw on her return: a woman physically identical to the one who married her son, but wholly absent.

'When I got back from Suffolk,' she says, 'you were gone.'

It is a typo. Not even a typo, in fact, but an unsteady hand. The nurse who had prepared our discharge summary had accidentally clicked on *palliative* instead of the correct word, directly above it on the drop-down menu, *paediatrics*. At discharge, Vida's specialism was paediatrics. It is as we thought. So we go back to the original uncertainty: what caused Vida's anaemia?

But it's too late to go back. I can no longer be measured, channel calm, expect the best. The unsteady hand has punctured that kind of optimism.

I flit between my hungry search for information and a desire to disappear. Some would call it a flight response, but I don't actively want to run away, to shirk my responsibilities, to cause anyone hurt. It's unconsciousness that I crave, to press pause on the unfolding of this difficult story – indefinitely. For the first time in my life, I forget about food entirely. While Freddie eats nervously, periodically stuffing pitta breads with hummus and chilli sauce, my eyes are glued either to my phone or to empty space. I feel relief at the opportunity to go to sleep each night, and dread at the prospect of being woken up so soon by Vida's hungry grunts. When she feeds on me in the darkness, I can feel what I might lose – and what I almost did.

We have a collection of words and numbers. Bone marrow. Severely anaemic. Haemoglobin. Reticulocytes.

We also have the facts, which I'm becoming practised at rattling off to new doctors in succinct headlines. I draw some satisfaction from exercising my brain for what feels like the first time in three months, but wish it were for some other reason. Vida was born at thirty-seven weeks and four days gestation by semi-emergency caesarean, with an HB of 115. Feeding started well and became progressively more difficult, her weight plateaued, then dropped just before she hit twelve weeks. She cried all the time, was listless, unhappy; she didn't like to sleep, nor really to be awake.

I look up some of the things that the doctors suggest could explain her anaemia. Instinctively, with no medical knowledge, I feel that some of them, such as the possibility of my mounting an immune response to her blood group, are not the culprits. In other cases, such as with parvovirus, I am hopeful that this episode is due to a bug I caught during pregnancy and will be something we can wash our hands of and leave behind. A quiver of foreboding tells me this might be too good to be true, too.

In searching 'severe anaemia 11 weeks baby', I fall upon a condition called Diamond-Blackfan anaemia. The words glint onscreen. What an extraordinary name, I think, almost Gothic, cultish. I click on it. Diamond-Blackfan anaemia (DBA) is an inherited bone-marrow failure syndrome, I learn, a blood disorder which primarily affects the body's ability to make red blood cells. Typically, babies decline into severe anaemia by two months of age, and diagnosis is most common at around four months. Vida is just over three months old.

My whole body reacts to what I read. My stomach churns, my fingers tingle. There's no denying that the condition bears striking resemblance to Vida's symptoms.

I read on. This Diamond-Blackfan thing has a differential diagnosis called transient erythroblastopenia of childhood (TEC). 'Transient' sounds promising. TEC initially presents in the same way as DBA, but after one or a maximum of two blood transfusions, healthy blood production starts up again. In comparing the two, one website describes DBA as 'grave', an unexpectedly emotive word for a medical paper.

Grave? I look at my pink and plump baby gurgling on the bed. She looks so well now. I put down my phone and pick her up to feed, imagining for a few wistful moments what it might be like to take her health at face value, pushing the twinkling of diamonds and waving of black fans to one side.

There is a scene in the first series of *Girls* in which Lena Dunham's character, Hannah – anxious in the way that we middle-class millennials specialise – googles 'diseases that come from no condom for one second' and then 'stuff that gets up around the sides of condoms', after having unprotected sex. At the time, it felt like seeing my own neuroses in action, and I cackled with laughter.

Dunham held up a mirror to a generation and specific group of women who had more choices and greater access to information than any before them. Women for whom the internet has been a kind of god, not the monotheistic kind our parents and grandparents grew up with, but one with millions of different authorities from which we could draw the conclusions we wanted. Was this search for knowledge a grappling for control? What was my use of Mumsnet when trying to conceive if not a symptom of the same thing?

I thought that if I knew what was going on, I could think my way out of whatever was blocking my path to happiness. I'd even been taught something along these lines when, a few years earlier, I'd started a reiki course and ended up sending good energy in the direction of friends and family all over the world, hoping that doing so might shift difficult challenges for them. Nothing was out of reach, nothing could not be wriggled away from.

And so, when Vida's anaemia is still unexplained two weeks after our admission, I turn to the place I rely on for answers. I go searching for reasons to believe the best. I develop a mental tally chart for DBA vs TEC, swinging between unease and hope like a pendulum multiple times a day.

Scientia potentia est. Knowledge is power. In the no-man's land of the undiagnosed, I learn a lot about blood very quickly in those early weeks, but knowledge presents too many possibilities to be empowering. Information becomes a reminder of my helplessness.

A diagnosis would be helpful, though. But while I want to know what is going on for Vida – 'the mercy of a name', as Anne Boyer describes it in her book *The Undying* – I am also fearful of answers. Perhaps because I have a sense that I'm not going to like them.

We visit Lewisham for a blood test twice a week. Each time, I notice that Freddie has put on a collared shirt and lace-up shoes. I wonder if these efforts are a superstition that he thinks might steer the course of things – a sartorial touching of wood? Or maybe on some level he thinks it will affect how seriously the doctors take him. Perhaps it is simply a kind of armour.

Every day we stare at our newly bonny baby in the north-facing light of the living room, hopeful with every successful feed and happy gurgle, willing her bone marrow into activity. I am reminded of that reiki course, sending energy from my fingertips to people who might need it, simply with the power of focused and positive thought. I wasn't ever sure I believed in it, but now my temples hurt from hoping it's real, that it works. Physically, too, I am sure there must be more I could do. Yes, I can love her, feed her, bathe her; and yes, I can comfort her, clothe her, sing to her. None of it feels enough. I want to be able to teach her how to make those blood cells, just as I might one day show her how to hold a fork. And failing that, I want to power her with my body, as I did for the thirty-seven weeks and four days until she was born. We may not share a bloodstream anymore, but I think about *The Two Fridas*, a painting by Frida Kahlo in which two versions of herself share a blood vessel, a lifeblood. If only I could do that. I am overcome with the desire to give my body up entirely to my daughter.

We are profoundly grateful to Lewisham for saving our daughter's life a couple of weeks ago, yet also frustrated. The paediatric doctors and nurses are always kind, but every time we go there we see someone different. Nobody seems to feel the same urgency as Freddie and me. I most probably need a target for my rage and, as the bearer of bad news, Lewisham Hospital is an easy one. It is time to push for that referral to the Evelina – we need a paediatric haematologist. We go to our GP prepared for a battle but are met by a kind clinician who quickly writes the letter. An appointment is made for a couple of weeks' time.

A fortnight shouldn't seem long, but the time stretches shapelessly ahead of us, empty of answers. I read and reread haematology articles and research papers on the likes of NCIH (National Centre for Complementary and Integrated Health) and blood.co.uk. Now when I search Vida's symptoms, the links are purple, not blue: old friends I revisit. In my old life, to reread something was a luxury; there was always something new to reroute my interests. Now, though, my mind is an echo chamber of blood, a haematology carousel. And though I've read them all before, each time I do so again, it is like the first time, a hungry appetite for information that might have changed into something more promising for us.

At night, I scroll away while Vida feeds back to sleep, her head supported by the crook of my elbow. Many precious moments pass like this, my fear illuminated by the light of my phone.

Our garden is growing in. We have abundant mint, oregano and sage in pots outside the kitchen, while purple-topped verbena stands tall in the flowerbeds, bobbing in the spring breeze like a Mexican wave. It had been a project, a rectangle of patchy lawn when we moved in, which we then filled with bulbs and troughs during the summer that Vida was conceived, with only an inkling of the shapes and colours that would emerge. Twelve months later, we have ourselves a little haven.

Despite this, we spend our days inside on the sofa – the BBC's coverage of the Chelsea Flower Show coddles us with Middle England's dahlias and Monty Don's utility wardrobe. Every few days we walk down to Lewisham Hospital for Vida's blood test, then wait for a phone call with her results. A full blood count (FBC) measures haemoglobin, also white blood cells, platelets and, when requested, reticulocytes, the young red blood cells that mature into vessels for haemoglobin. So far, all of Vida's white blood cell and platelet counts have come back normal. She held her haemoglobin well for a few days after the first transfusion, but it is now trending down again. This is bad news. On one occasion, though, we see some uplift in reticulocytes. I experience this kernel of hope like pure oxygen.

But we are ragged. I lean heavily on Freddie, and he in turn leans heavily on our mothers. My mum, who lives twenty-five minutes away, pops in on weekdays; his mum lives north of the river and comes for the weekends. When they leave, everything takes on a blurred quality, uncontained by a routine of hot meals and parental optimism.

I have also built up difficult associations with our home. The flat has been the setting for many days spent on my own with Vida, with Freddie back at work – days of failed feeds, clock-watching, and pained looks from the dog. Days of willing Freddie to walk through the front door. This is where Vida grew really sick, where a GP missed her anaemia, where I'd not acted on instinct and pushed for help, where she'd ultimately been admitted for life-saving treatment. It is not an easy place to be.

We are comfortable at Louise's house. We'd spent the early part of our relationship living with her while we saved for our first home. For Freddie, Louise offers support that perhaps only a mother can; I am bolstered by her pragmatism and drawn to the light that her experience can shed. She lost her parents young and raised Freddie on her own. She is no stranger to uphill struggles but is one of the most dependable people I know: wise, fun and accomplished – living proof that some people can not only survive hard times, they can thrive.

Her house, a terrace in West Hampstead, is where Freddie grew up. It has been the setting for thirty years of undulating family life, and of therapy between Louise and her patients. This house is expert at containing turmoil, at helping to resolve crises. It feels safe and it feels known. I know the squeaks of its hinges, the slam of its kitchen door; I know that Louise's schedule means I must hide on the hour and at ten minutes to the next one to avoid seeing a patient; I know that Freddie will come home at 6.05 p.m. because his studio is just around the corner. In this time of uncertainty, the value of what is known has never been higher.

So we pack bags of clothes and baby clobber and leave our flat for NW6 with all its familiarity and certainty. I have nothing to prove here. And, crucially, I know no one with a baby.

The day has come for our appointment with Dr Alamelu at the Evelina. My mum joins us, as has become the norm. She has taken to the situation like the investigative reporter she trained to be (note-taking, reading, speaking to doctor friends), but I can sense that she is as shit-scared as I am. The cakes flow daily – diversion baking – and she has adopted a mantra: Vida's symptoms must have been 'a freak anomaly', not a sign of serious disease.

We meet at Blackfriars station and we walk along the river towards St Thomas' Hospital. It is early summer and the city is starting to bare its skin. Outside the British Film Institute people peruse second-hand books and drink lunchtime rosé while children watch the street performers, entranced. An accordion plays and new mums sit together beside the National Theatre with their buggies and keep-cups. Tourists queue for the London Eye, where the air is heavy with the scent of sugary chocolate sauce and lager. We walk past it all.

Evelina is the Guy's and St Thomas' (GSTT) specialist children's hospital. Just across the river from the Houses of Parliament, GSTT is Britain's biggest hospital trust, comprising Guy's in London Bridge and St Thomas' in Lambeth. Evelina has its own building, a tall, light-filled glass structure, connected to St Thomas' via an umbilical corridor. Standing in its foyer, I have the sense of being a part of something big, powerful, nurturing. Surrounding us now is a din of excitable children and energised staff, not to mention bursts of colour with murals, toys and a giant helter-skelter. It is a stimulating space for kids (Vida will one day ride its glass lift with much enthusiasm) and a relatively uplifting one for addled parents. Each floor is named after a different ecosystem, and each area on that floor after a creature that might live in it (the haemophilia and thrombosis office, for example, is in 'Puffin' on 'Ocean').

The Evelina feels like somewhere that advances are made, and important things happen. I can see how much thought has gone into the function and use of this space. Strategy like this requires funding. The manga cartoons along the corridors, picturing a group of characters I will later learn are called the 'Evelina gang', are triply reassuring to me: I know they appeal to children, softening the edges of somewhere in which hard things happen; they help us to find our way in a place prone to overwhelming the already overwhelmed, and they suggest budget. In reception, I look up and see, on the walls of the first floor, a list of high-profile donors. (This is probably the first and last time I will feel grateful to McDonald's.)

Dr Alamelu is softly spoken and calming, priceless qualities in a busy hospital. Vida seems less of a mystery to her than to the general paediatricians we've seen, even if the problem remains unsolved. We talk through all the events to date and she encourages us to stay hopeful – it could be a transient anaemia. My lungs fill with relief; it feels as though I haven't breathed this deeply in weeks. She says she'll run more blood tests, throwing in one for Diamond-Blackfan anaemia on the off-chance. She seems happy with the plucky baby girl on my lap, with her comedy quiff of hair and dewy eyes, which I've noticed are starting to turn more green. I take another deep breath.

I'm learning quickly, though, that haematology requires a lot of watching and waiting and, once more, we are told we must wait: this time, for today's blood results. In the meantime, we must continue doing what we're doing and keep an eye on her. 'Just enjoy your baby,' says one of the nurses, seeing my stricken expression. Like many people who do her job, she really cares, she wants to help, so she doesn't deserve to be told how absolutely fucking hard it is to 'just enjoy' our baby while high-stake question marks hang over us.

Having psyched myself up for a more conclusive end to this consultation, I feel deflated by this return to limbo. We walk back to the station quiet, shaky, blank. I have Vida asleep in the sling on my chest, oblivious to the storm inside it.

On the platform, Mum misses her train as I start to cry. She holds my hand in one of hers, Freddie's in the other.

'Listen,' she says, her voice breaking, 'the only thing you can do right now . . . all you have to do is *love* this little baby with everything you have.'

She strokes the wave of chestnut hair crowning Vida's head, kisses us both and sees us onto our train. She waves as it pulls out of the station, not moving until we are out of sight. All I can think is that I want my mummy.

The weeks pass at a snail's pace. I flit between purposeful googling and a breathless feeling of impotence. Everything and nothing hurts, worry transposed into unspecific pain. When I develop a lump on my left arm, I become convinced it is something sinister, but there is perverse relief in the distraction it brings. It is on the side of my radius bone, right where Vida's head is positioned when she feeds on my left side; it hurts sharply when she moves. I go to the doctor who suspects it is a ganglion cyst, possibly caused by a bruise and exacerbated by the baby's feeding. Once I hear this, it quickly heals.

I never have the opportunity of a night to catch up after broken sleep; this is of course true for most new parents, but this kind of exhaustion blocks rational thought right when I need it most. Freddie is brilliant at taking Vida in the mornings, and I am loath to ask more of him in the middle of the night, knowing how much I rely on him right now, his steadiness made possible in part by rest. The early days of crunching through granola while Vida fed in the small hours – an adventure in sleeplessness made cuter by fairy lights and snacks – are over now. Nowadays I sit up in bed and nurse her in the dark, my stomach too preoccupied to rumble.

No sooner than we had met with Dr Alamelu at the Evelina, I start to notice changes in Vida. The zeal with which she took to feeding after her first transfusion is giving way to a fussiness I recognise. She whinges, seemingly for food, but when I offer her a feed, she shakes her head, eyes squeezed shut, crying gummily as if to say, *You're not hearing me.*

I analyse her colour, her nappies, her feeding. The Saturday after our appointment, we go to my parents' for lunch. I am particularly bad when I'm with my mum and dad, feeling permission, perhaps, for my terror to boil over. At lunch, Vida cries a lot in my arms. It's impossible to eat but my appetite left the building a while ago. Mum, always confident in the restorative effect of a dog walk, suggests the two of us take her to the park.

Predictably, the baby conks out to the motion of the pram. Streatham Common is buxom in its June dress. The horse-chestnut candelabras are out, neon-pink-flecked, and green blackberries have started to dot the brambles. We have been walking here since I was a little girl; it feels like a foundation of my psychic geography, although I feel none of its grounding qualities now. Mum is talking to me about staying positive, but I hear her only distantly. I look at my daughter's sleeping face. She is pale. The tiny purple blood vessels around her closed eyes sit in high contrast to her complexion, and I'm sure her lips are a lighter pink than they were a couple of weeks ago. Fresh blood had given her a look of pudginess you expect in a baby of four months old, but today I notice she has lost that definition.

I am more conscious of my instinct now. Even if I don't like what it is telling me, I have promised myself not to be talked out of it like before. I am also conscious of how much time has passed since our stint at Lewisham: almost four weeks. I know from my reading that with transient anaemias, one transfusion alone is usually enough to set a child back on the path to producing their own red blood cells. Children with Diamond-Blackfan anaemia, on the other hand, require blood transfusions every three to four weeks in order to maintain a healthy haemoglobin level. With Vida starting to look pale again, DBA wins a point. My head swims with all this haematology knowledge that is both basic and highly specialised, and that sense of foreboding returns.

Mum suggests going to church. She wonders if it might help me to find a place of peace. I am aware of people who rely on faith to see them through times like this and of others who find it. I am neither of these, it turns out.

Religion had been a faint metronome in my childhood: Easter, Christmas, Brownies at our local London church, the Lord's Prayer in school assembly, notions of heaven as a reward and hell as a threat. Later, I got married in a church, insisting, of course, on replacing the 'obey' in my set of vows, also troubled by the presence of only our fathers' professions on the marriage certificate. But the church itself – Salthouse, on the north Norfolk coast – is an incredible, sparse space beside my dad's childhood home, and where Freddie's dad Charlie's funeral had been held seven years earlier. On some level, we felt spiritually connected to the place. November light flooded in through the north window, and afterwards several people said they had felt that Charlie was there in spirit. I could feel my grannies there, too – Jane singing 'Tell Out My Soul' with gusto, while Mavis (looking spectacular in her best magenta coat) burrowed through her handbag for some collection coins.

Faith, then, was something I had dipped into when it suited me. I belonged to the Church of England by inheritance. I thought the Bible contained important values and lessons, but also plenty that were questionable. Its characters felt remote, its stories abstract. I lived a good – and, I thought, kind – life without church and enjoyed a service at Christmas for nostalgia's sake.

But the last few weeks in and out of hospitals have brought home our biology to me. I have never been more conscious that I am little more than an assembly of cells. Religion seems incompatible with science. I just don't see how they can coexist, though I know many doctors are believers.

However, I am conflicted. I want the faith that will let me believe that Vida can beat this. Over the course of my school years, assemblies had segued from hymns and Christian prayers to non-denominational, secular invocations, but I'd long since absorbed God-fearing by osmosis. I had worried that if I said I didn't believe out loud, something awful might happen.

I wrestle with the idea of there being a reason for what's happened to Vida. Had we done something to deserve this? Did I invite it with my frantic efforts to get pregnant, or with the unmotherly thoughts I'd had when we wondered if Vida was simply difficult, rather than unwell? And why us?

Guilt tugs at me whenever I have these thoughts. I feel grateful not just to have a baby, but to have *this* baby, this little girl who, when she feels well, has the greatest smile. It's a smile I recognise – like someone I have known for a long time, I know her deeply. And I am absolutely hers. I delight in her concentrated frown as she kicks her legs when we change her nappy; her funny Tintin quiff; the way she sucks hungrily on my chin, mistaking it for a boob; how she responds to music, in which her taste runs the gamut of nursery rhymes to Major Lazer. After the first transfusion, I could look at her and see no visible illness. It is easy to imagine the problem away.

Despite dismissing Mum's suggestion of church, Freddie and I do start praying. While Vida sleeps, swaddled next to us, we sit on our knees, facing the wall in the dark, and hold our hands together in prayer. Freddie says he would like to start, 'Dear Lord,' he says, 'please help us and our baby.'

'Please spare her from Diamond-Blackfan anaemia,' I chime in, cutting to the chase. I make no bones with God.

Weekends are an endurance. Two full days when health services are harder to access, forty-eight whole hours when we definitely won't hear from a hospital with Vida's blood results. In this way, I'm already becoming institutionalised. I resent being in the hospital when we're there, but I'm on edge when we're not.

On the Monday after lunch with my parents, I meet Dad at a gallery. I imagine this situation would be challenging for any parent, not least for a man who is so solutions-oriented. He has always loved fixing things. But the current state of affairs precludes me or Vida from being fixed because we don't know what we're dealing with.

Galleries, though, Dad can do. Over the summer, he, Vida and I do lots of the things I'd imagined we would during my maternity leave, which has coordinated with his retirement. It feels nothing like I hoped it would, more of a consolation prize for a difficult few months than a revelling in intergenerational cultural experience, but my dad's version of support – not so much talking but *doing* – feels poignant; he battles with arthritic knees to schlep around London with me and Vida. We see a show about 1930s printmaking at the Dulwich Picture Gallery, visit Karl Marx's grave in Highgate (Dad has become a communist and is reading *Das Kapital* for the third time), and regularly do the rounds of London's two Tate galleries. And there's always a café visit. I suspect he is sent out under instruction from Mum to make sure I eat. Today we are at the Tate Modern and he has loaded up a tray. His approach to getting food into me is less subtle or strategic than Mum's – 'Come on, eat something,' the pushing of a sandwich towards me – and his directness makes me want to try. But food has lost its taste; it sits uncomfortably in my stomach.

I want to be wrong, but I am sure Vida is anaemic again. Before meeting Dad, I'd called Dr Alamelu's secretary, desperate for her to tell me what to do. She had been in clinic. Now we sit in the Tate Modern members' room. Two jolly women are at the neighbouring table, giddy on lunchtime wine. They coo as I lift Vida from the pram, fiddle with the hook on my bra, bring her to my chest. She shakes her head and bawls, and the women quickly look away, recharging their glasses. Suddenly, my phone rings and I hear Dr Alamelu's gentle voice, 'Hello, is that Vida's mum?'

I tell her the latest – the failed feeds, the crying, how I think her pallor has come back. We are due a blood test in three days' time, but, she says, 'If she were mine, I think I'd bring her in sooner.' This is as clear an instruction as I could get from her. I abandon an untouched tuna mayo on granary, give my dad a kiss, and walk down the South Bank to St Thomas', where more blood is taken from Vida while I sob.

Dr Alamelu calls again late in the afternoon. Vida's haemoglobin has fallen to 78 over four weeks.

We are booked into the Evelina for a blood transfusion the following day.

The second transfusion of Vida's life has been arranged by the lead specialist nurse at the Evelina Hospital's Haemophilia and Thrombosis Centre. As a child with a suspected blood disorder, her care falls under them, despite the fact that both haemophilia and thrombosis are clotting disorders. It's an anomaly, which illustrates how unusual cases like Vida's are.

The nurse is brisk and kind, at pains to tell me that their other patient with DBA – if that's what Vida has – leads a 'completely normal life'. I bristle when I hear that this world centre in paediatrics has only one other patient. It is so rare. I say that a blood transfusion every three weeks doesn't sound very normal to me.

We have lost track of how many days Freddie has taken off work since Vida was born. Luckily, he is self-employed and his best friend, Joe, happens to be his business partner. Going back to work has offered him distraction and relief from the chaos at home, most of all from me. I'm conscious that caring for Vida and having my own feelings is taking all the fight I have and that I am not reciprocating his support. The person he married isn't really there; just her body – and a changed body, too. Clothes hang off me in a way I would have been pleased by in the past. I subsist on a diet of pastry and caffeine. Every morning, Freddie takes Vida from me at 6 a.m. and, while I sleep, he pushes her up to Hampstead, returning with a coffee and a croissant for me.

On that first day at the Evelina, I wear trainers, a pair of dark pink tracksuit bottoms and a light pink feeding vest with spaghetti straps. In a few months' time, I will read a short story by Lorrie Moore, which takes place on a children's ward, describing the mothers with 'their blond hair and sweatpants and sneakers and determined pleasantness'. Clearly I have the uniform down from day one; less so the demeanour. I have seen that shrill cheeriness on Facebook parent groups.

We walk down the wide corridor of St Thomas'. Mounted on the walls are pictures of Victorian nursery rhymes painted onto tiles, a gift to the hospital from Doulton's of Lambeth pottery in the early twentieth century: Little Bo Peep, Little Jack Horner, Little Miss Muffet – blonde, blue-eyed specimens in an England of yore. I can't help but imagine lines and blood bags attached to all of them.

At the end of the corridor is a lift, which takes us to our destination on the first floor: Snow Fox. We ring a bell and are buzzed into a ward flooded with natural light. I am struck by its colour and bustle. Cartoon foxes scurry down the corridor walls, and above each bed is an illustrated plaque that playfully spells out the bed's number. Even the ceiling tiles have pictures on them. The paediatric ward at Lewisham mirrored my bleakness back at me; this place does the opposite. The vibe is positively upbeat.

We are greeted with the smiles of a woman in blue scrubs; her name badge says Hana. She shows us to our bay, where a shiny new cot, bright green and blue, sits beneath an illustrated bedhead. She offers us tea, strokes Vida's hair, wheels in a giant illuminating sensory toy and a blood-pressure monitor to start some observations. I understand the significance of today, of a second transfusion, of what this could mean for Vida's diagnosis. It weighs heavy, but I feel held by this place and its people.

A nurse in darker blue scrubs comes over and introduces himself as Patrick. He turns to Vida, who takes his finger in a chubby grip and waves it up and down, her eyes crossing as they follow the motion of their held hands. 'Hello bubba,' he says to her. Vida started smiling a few weeks ago, before her first admission – miraculously, because she can't have felt much like smiling then. She holds Patrick's gaze intently, not smiling exactly, but intrigued and at peace. Between Freddie and me, there is a sense of unspoken surprise.

We learn that Snow Fox was renovated less than a year ago and quietly remark to each other about the difference it makes to us. I worry that it seems a bit superficial to have had this thought – it doesn't matter what the ward looks like so long as Vida is getting the treatment she needs – but Freddie disagrees. Anything that makes it easier is to be celebrated, he says.

It matters how hospitals look. Good design and thoughtful use of art are uplifting, but also subtly say to patients and caregivers, 'We've thought about you; you matter.'

Snow Fox is a day unit for paediatric outpatients, serving children who need routine treatments to keep them well, such as blood transfusions and infusions of medicines. Cannulating small veins is a speciality here. Patrick comes over with some little boxes and a stack of large, clear plasters. He tells us that he's going to apply a numbing cream to help make the cannula less painful for Vida. We've never heard of numbing cream before. I teeter between feeling grateful that it exists and fury that this is the first I've heard of it. It takes forty-five minutes to work, he says, dabbing it onto her hands, elbows, feet, then sticking the plasters over.

Vida whinges as the cold cream is applied. She is due a nap and I go to lie on the bed, unhooking my bra, ready for the familiar tussle. But she latches on, sucking a couple of times before her mouth loosens and her tracing-paper eyelids close. Hana comes and tucks a pillow under her, bringing her closer to my body. Then she tilts the bed upright with a remote control; I let it take my weight and my spine and head sink back. Cradling Vida, I am cradled.

In the past I would have charted London according to food and drink. Give me a postcode, and I'd point you towards a good meal. The Knowledge for the greedy. If I'd had reason to come to St Thomas', I would have gone to the coffee roastery on Lower Marsh if it was the morning, or schlepped to the Anchor and Hope at lunchtime, or to the Garden Museum

Café for a cake in the afternoon. I understood the capital's topography in edible terms. These things don't occur to me now. Instead, I am zealously filling my mind with medicine: 50 per cent haematology, to second-guess what is going on in my daughter's body, and 50 per cent genetics, to understand what could have caused all this, and how it might be remedied.

I reason that I am preparing myself for the worst to soften the blow if and when it comes. And I can't think about anything else. I am possessed by the condition, going mad with its possibility, like the doomed protagonist in a Gothic novel. Diamond-Blackfan anaemia certainly sounds like a fitting name, conjuring fear, darkness. I imagine crows encircling us and stealing my baby in their talons.

Each human contains around 20,000 genes. They come in pairs, one copy from each parent. DBA is an autosomal dominant condition: this means that only one of those two parental genes needs to be mutated for a baby to have it. So, if Vida has DBA, just one of the two cells from which she originated – the sperm and the egg – would have carried a faulty copy of the gene. The majority of cases of DBA are *de novo*, or 'anew', caused by a spontaneous mutation, meaning that neither parent has it. In some cases, however, an asymptomatic parent finds out that they have DBA after their child has been diagnosed. It's also possible for one parent to carry the mutation in some of their eggs or sperm cells.

There are a number of mutations associated with DBA and almost innumerable ways that they can be expressed physically. An inability to produce red blood cells is the severest and most common symptom but by no means the only one. There are patients with congenital anomalies – skeletal issues in the spine, triangulated thumbs (an anomaly where the thumbs have three joints instead of two) or genital disfigurement; some are deaf, others have heart abnormalities. Some patients are already anaemic *in utero*; others become so within their first few months; some suddenly and inexplicably become anaemic after years of life; others still get by on a low but manageable haemoglobin level their entire lives. Some respond to steroid treatment incredibly well, freeing them from the need for transfusions; others remain transfusion-dependent; others still require a bone-marrow transplant. I learn that some families never find out their child's mutation and that not all the genetic causes of DBA have been discovered yet. It is a labyrinthine condition with many pathways.

The more I read about it, the more I fear it. But it's already too late for blissful ignorance. I've always believed that knowledge is power and I have never felt so powerless. My head reels with what it could mean for Vida if she has DBA; with the chance that Freddie or I might have it; with the odds of our future children having it. There is so much to take on board. So much variation between cases. So many ifs and buts and maybes. The big question mark of whether Vida has it at all.

It takes three nurses and two parents to cannulate Vida. To hold her arm; to insert the line, then quickly secure it with a teddy-bear plaster; to attach a splint and bandage it around her arm, which holds it in place during a transfusion; to soothe her cries with rattles (Freddie) and breastmilk (me). They have put the cannula in her elbow because I've been assertive about wanting to avoid her hands, if possible. They are still bruised, nearly five weeks on from her admission to Lewisham.

Unfortunately, we learn, elbows are tricky because they bend and can cause a blockage in the line, an occlusion. However, deft and calm, Patrick makes the difficult process of cannulating Vida seem simple. He points, aims and withdraws the needle, and her distress is minimised. But she always cries and we always emerge shaken up. When Vida is ready in her fresh lint boxing glove, it feels like we've already been in a fight. I begin to feed her and look over at Freddie. I feel for him. Much as I may have felt tethered by the demands of breastfeeding, it is as comforting to me as it is to Vida when she is upset; he doesn't have that. I can only imagine how impotent he feels.

Most of my friends feel very far away – and not as the crow flies. Many of them don't have children, and if I'd already felt anxious about how motherhood might have changed me, recent events have made much of my old life feel very remote. I feel I have nothing to offer people and so avoid them, leaving many messages not just unanswered but unread. I don't want to field their sympathetic looks when I tell them about the hospital visits, or their kind attempts to follow when I explain the situation with my new medical vocabulary.

Equally, I don't enjoy telling the story out loud, reliving and making more real the previously unthinkable.

Worst of all is when people tell me they're sure she'll be OK. It recalls the affirmations I remember from our hypnobirthing classes and the intentions I used to set before having a massage, which taught that my mind had the power to shape a sequence of events. When one person tells us that she'll be fine because they 'feel it in their bones', I am conflicted, reassured by their strength of belief, and incensed by its naivety. *HOW DO YOU FUCKING KNOW?* I want to scream. The power of positive thinking has never felt so irrelevant – it can't undo a medical condition if Vida has it. There's no spiritual bypass for this.

Even Freddie feels distant, with his calm in the face of my frenzy and his soft snores at night. How is he sleeping? Eating? Going to work? I hear him enthuse about food or take work calls, nimbly switching in and out of personae when I can only inhabit my sadness. I am lonely and want to be less so, but am only open to a certain kind of company. The handful of friends that I am in touch with have inhabited what Susan Sontag called the Kingdom of the Sick. All of us will at some point belong to that kingdom, will have 'this more onerous citizenship', as well as one to the kingdom of the well. Sickness is a universal threat – it can and will strike us all. But in the summer of 2019, I feel alone with my family in the more onerous citizenship. I am in my early thirties and most of my friends are still enjoying the good passport, although a couple know that other place, of hospitals and of uncertainty: my school friend Beatrice, whose mum has been battling with ill health for years; my NCT friend Boo, an oncology nurse. Both know what to say to me. Both realise the seriousness. Both see that I don't want distraction but to look at it in the face. They do so with me.

I've also started scouring the web for other people's stories about their ill children. I've already read all the individual DBA stories that I can find – mostly tabloid articles designed to tug at the heart strings and raise funds, saying things like 'no cure' and 'their only hope'. I am interested in these stories, in other people's pain and how they have handled it, and I've stopped being fussy about the conditions I read about now – cancers, dystrophies, other blood disorders – if they can show me a way to cope.

Once or twice, I use the preposterous search term 'celebrities with sick kids'. I want to know about people who seem to thrive in spite of tragedy, and what better examples, I think, than those with public lives, the rich and famous?

Gary Lineker's son recovered from leukaemia.

Colin Farrell's son lives with a rare genetic disorder.

Gordon Brown and David Cameron both lost children to illness.

I am moved by what I find. The vulnerability of parenthood is a great equaliser.

It dawns on me that while my daughter *might* have a rare blood condition, she *definitely* has the human condition.

And we all have that.

The Kingdom of the Sick lurks there for us all.

Back on Snow Fox, and Vida's transfusion has started. As her system fills with haemoglobin, she perks up. When she is awake it is tricky to keep her arm still. When the line occludes, usually because it is kinked, the transfusion automatically stops, setting off an alarm, and Patrick or Hana scurry in to reset it.

Freddie and I take it in turns to hold her so that the other can enjoy some hands-free time. During his, Freddie has discovered a food market in the garden in front of St Thomas' and comes back to the ward happily brandishing wraps and mezze boxes. During mine, I pick up my phone. In the past I would have opened Instagram on autopilot and scrolled dumbly through my feed, but I deleted it last month, offended by its curated take on life and, specifically, the easy passage into parenthood that some of my contemporaries seemed to be experiencing. Now I go nervously to open Safari, all ready to read and reread medical articles and parent testimonies. But Beatrice has messaged me.

Did you know that a food and drink editor of the FT has a son with DBA?

I didn't. She sends me the link to 'How I came to love the NHS', an article published six months ago by journalist Alexander Gilmour, who, I am incredulous to discover, is indeed a food editor at the *Financial Times*. The piece details his son's difficult birth, an eventual diagnosis with Diamond-Blackfan anaemia and his profound gratitude for the institution that has been taking care of him.

I can hardly believe it. *Five to seven in a million live births worldwide.*

I email him immediately.

Only the genetic test can definitively tell us what we're dealing with — assuming, that is, that if Vida has Diamond-Blackfan, she has a recognised mutation.

I've been told that her genetic results will take an absolute minimum of six weeks, but that doesn't stop me hoping they might come sooner. I make regular calls to the geneticist at Guy's and to Dr Alamelu's secretary. My education made sure I was proficient in the art of polite pressure. It has always worked for me.

But this is not a question of getting a refund or securing a restaurant reservation. Nobody cares about my sensitively crafted, grammatical emails or the *Guardian* logo in my email signature. The system is the system. I am just another patient's parent. I learn as much about my privilege as I do about medicine in these weeks.

That night, when we are home from the transfusion with Vida, newly pink and hungry, Alexander Gilmour emails me back. His words are warm and I feel a tingle of kinship instantly. 'I have a thousand things to tell you,' he says. 'I think we should meet.' We arrange to do so the following week.

I have never met Alexander Gilmour but I recognise him from his Twitter avatar. I have looked at the image a lot over the weekend, studying it for traces of what he has been through. It is strange to have so much in common – food, newspapers, London – and to plan to touch on none of it. Only the other thing.

We go to a café and I shift vegan burger around my mouth while he tells me some of his family's story. I hear his fluency with words that are gradually becoming part of my vernacular: steroids, cannulas, haemoglobin. I can't be easy lunch company, unable to hide my horror at the condition that his child has. But I get the impression that Alexander, or rather, Al, feels some relief to meet someone – a stranger, yes, but still, a person from his world – who knows something about all this, the blood talk and fear that characterised his first year as a father. Al has learnt that DBA is so rare and so complex that even the most decorated paediatric haematologist at the most prestigious children's hospital is unlikely to have the knowledge to offer patients the right care. If Vida's genetic test results come back positive for DBA, he tells me, we must push for a referral to a doctor he mentioned in his first email, Dr Josu de la Fuente. He is the country's only specialist in the condition.

Given how my feelings about religion have evolved recently, I am briefly tickled by the name Josu: Basque for Jesus. Maybe *this* Jesus, Dr Jesus, can help us.

I have been doing more reading about treatments for Diamond-Blackfan anaemia. Most parents seem to hope that steroids will work. The idea is that every child with a confirmed diagnosis tries prednisolone, a steroid drug, initially at a high dose, in the hope that their bone marrow will be jolted into producing red blood cells. If the child responds well, the dose is tapered down slowly so that they take an almost 'homeopathic' amount every other day for the rest of their lives. Given this means they no longer need blood transfusions, it seems like a good outcome, but it only works for about 30 per cent of patients. And even then, there is always the risk that their bone marrow might relapse (this often happens during puberty, for example). Lifelong medical supervision remains a must.

My mum – who took prednisolone while recovering from pneumonia when I was a child – waxes lyrical about how 'turbo-charged' she felt on it. I remember her scurrying around like Sonic the Hedgehog at six o'clock in the morning; steroid treatment had an almost magical effect on her health and, used for short periods, offers many patients with various ailments a miracle cure. But, long-term, steroids can be problematic. DBA is the only condition for which lifelong steroid treatment is used, and with it can come a host of complications, from slowed growth to osteoporosis, weight gain, trouble sleeping and mental health problems.

I hate the sound of steroids. I also hate the idea of lifelong blood transfusions. And, even more, I hate the prospect of chelation, the treatment which offsets the iron build-up caused by transfusions. Some patients can take a pill called Exjade, but if their liver doesn't tolerate it, they are put on Desferal, a drug given by subcutaneous injection overnight. Parents have to administer this, sticking a needle into their child's leg every bedtime.

Al had told me that for his son, he was rooting for gene therapy, even though this was a treatment not yet available – and might not be for another fifteen years or so, maybe even longer, considering DBA's rareness. It would be the closest thing to a fix but at this point seems too abstract to bank on.

Bone-marrow transplants (BMT) are divisive in the DBA community, but I am drawn to the idea. BMT replaces the child's faulty bone marrow with that of a matched donor so that they are haematologically cured: no more blood transfusions, no worry about steroids failing, no waiting around for elusive gene therapy.

Though I know it is naive, I become convinced that, if Vida has DBA, her best option will be a transplant. I don't want illness to be her life's focus. I want her to have all the freedom of movement and mind that healthy children and adults have. If that means we spend a year in isolation first, so be it. If that means chemotherapy for Vida, we can do it. I ignore the possibility of serious complications in my belief that we'd battle through it and emerge triumphant. Mostly, I am buoyed by the fact that there is something we can actively do to address Vida's problem if necessary.

The better the donor match, the better the chances of the transplant working. The gold standard here is to have a sibling donor. Some families already have another child whose stem cells match their affected sibling's, just by chance – the probability of this happening is 25 per cent – but others set out to create one, using a specialised form of IVF called pre-implantation genetic diagnosis (PGD). Once embryos have been created with eggs and sperm, their stem-cell profiles are tested to see if any of them match that of their sibling.

I read about families who have undergone this lengthy process and ended up with a successful bone-marrow transplant. One couple has a daughter with DBA who was successfully transplanted with the bone marrow of a sister conceived in this way. They kept a blog during the process, with photos not only of what was clearly a difficult few months in hospital, but also of their kids playing in bubble baths, on bikes, in parks, enjoying the hallmarks of happy family life in spite of DBA.

Even without a diagnosis, I find myself searching for kernels of hope, looking for fixes, for ways out of this for her. For now, the idea of BMT offers me the purpose I need. IVF, I decide, is what we will do if Vida is diagnosed. And helplessness gives way to purpose.

—

It is the end of June and we are back at the Evelina's Haemophilia and Thrombosis Centre. Weekly blood tests since Vida's first transfusion at Snow Fox have shown that her haemoglobin is in decline again. A nurse has just drawn another sample, and Vida is upset. I'm realising her resistance to needles is less about pain than it is about constraint. She arches her back, kicks her legs, waves her arms; I hold her on my lap, facing outwards, catching flailing limbs and holding her in position. This amplifies her screams. Our combined heart rate must be off the chart.

Dr Alamelu peers around the door: she has news. One of the results from a previous test, which looked at the level of an enzyme called eADA in Vida's blood, is back. Her reading is double the upper limit of normal. While a raised eADA is not a diagnosis, there is a known connection between this and DBA. She had thought that Vida's anaemia wasn't due to DBA in our first meeting; now she is less sure.

I ask her if Diamond-Blackfan is now looking more likely.

She shifts her weight, clenches her jaw a little. 'Yes,' she says quietly, 'but let's wait for the genetics before drawing that conclusion.'

Vida has now recovered from her blood test and is gurgling at a halogen light on the ceiling. I hug her to me, breathe in her sweet cereal-milk hair, exhale, determined not to cry.

'Well, this is shit,' I spit.

The room falls silent. Freddie elbows me. 'That's not helpful,' he says, under his breath.

—

Hospitals are not easy places for Freddie. When he was only twenty, his dad died after three months in hospital as the result of a devastating accident.

And hospitals have proved a distinguishing feature of Freddie's experience of being a father, too: my series of mysterious scans in late pregnancy, the drama of Vida's birth, followed by the heart-murmur kerfuffle. Then the emergency blood transfusion, the continued anaemia, now this interminable wait for a diagnosis. The people he loves don't usually emerge from hospital cured or with clear answers.

Nonetheless, he makes a valiant effort to keep our spirits up. Maybe he has no choice. He throws himself into restoring order to our lives in whatever ways he can. It's all important grown-up stuff, but, in my eyes, frivolous. Meal planning! Redecorating! A new car!

The square meal we've cooked every evening since forever has suddenly fallen to him and his mum. I find myself pushing morsels around my plate until we clear up. He has organised for two bedrooms in Louise's house – one for us, one for Vida – to be redecorated because he feels keenly that nice spaces bring calm. And he is excited about the family-sized vehicle he's decided to lease. I know I have to muster some interest in it, not least because I'm giving him so little else at the moment.

We walk through West Hampstead to the dealership to finalise some of the details. A buggy passes us; I study the colour of the child within it – ginger hair and bright white skin against a dark anorak. I don't understand why Vida's colour is 'pallor', a sign of illness, while this kid just gets to be 'pale'.

'Do you think it's going to be DBA?' I ask him as he strides along with the pram, 'Or do you think we will move on from this?' My questions are direct these days, no British prancing around them.

I no longer trust people's good instincts about what will unfold, but I still cast around for reassurance. I want Freddie to tell me that no, he thinks this will pass, that this heartache will have all the transience of a bad breakup, eventually fading into the trace of a scar on the skin of our shared history.

'It probably is,' he replies. 'You don't expect someone who keeps beating you up to suddenly give you flowers, do you?'

June gives way to July. Three weeks after our first visit to Snow Fox, we are back for another transfusion. Dr Alamelu comes to our bay to tell us in person.

Vida has Diamond-Blackfan anaemia.

Of diagnosis, Anne Boyer writes, 'Now you don't have a solution to a problem, now you have a specific name for a life breaking in two.'

I feel it snap.

I am twirling a bamboo spoon in the air, trying to catch Vida's eye. The spoon holds a tiny mouthful of sweet potato, bright orange and caramelised at the edges from slightly too long in the oven. I had long been planning to make this her first meal, anticipating her green eyes light up at something tasting this good. But she's not the slightest bit interested in my orange aeroplane, preferring the mobile of black-and-white stuffed houses dangling above her vibrating chair.

This baby puts everything in her mouth except, it seems, food. She won't open it for the spoon, and when I give it to her to hold, she shakes it, looks at it quizzically, drops it, then turns her attention back to the mobile. She is nineteen weeks old, so we are a good few weeks away from the recommended age to start weaning, six months.

I've talked myself into trying her on solids sooner for several reasons. Out loud, I say that I'm overwhelmed by the pressures of being a human dairy. Now that it's working well, I actually love breastfeeding but, ever since her weight started to drop before we went into Lewisham, feeding her has been a constant source of worry. I find not knowing how much of my milk she's had stressful, and she won't take a bottle. Perhaps the Technicolor world of flavour will seduce her to eating more, and in ways that I can measure? And maybe this, in turn, will make for fewer disrupted nights?

Eventually, I manage to get a little mound of sweet potato onto her tongue. She frowns, squints, pouts and spits it out with impressive force.

I find the strength of my daughter's mind reassuring given what we now know about her health. But it's also a head-fuck. The smiling, the cooing, the obnoxious rejection of orange mush is hardly the image of an unwell baby. I can't reconcile what I'm seeing with the gravity of the diagnosis.

I am ready to fight for Vida to have the most and the best of everything: love, food, medical care. I'll wean her, I think, on strength-enhancing green things – spinach, like Popeye, or baby guacamole, in tribute to *The Avocado Baby*, John Burningham's story around a weak baby that grows strong on a diet of avocados. But then, suddenly, I will feel defeated. All the good food in the world can't change the condition.

I know I let her down when I have these thoughts. I am trying hard for her not to see me upset, reserving that for Freddie and our parents when she is asleep. (Lucky them.)

Sometimes my sadness becomes too much to bear. When I

hand Vida to one of the others, so I can go to the loo or, luxury of luxuries, have a shower, I feel dizzy with the freedom but quickly bereft. If I hear her crying and am not in the same room, I go to her, look her in the eyes, calm her. This comforts me as much as it does her: we want each other. She stops crying in my arms, grunts happily when she feeds from me.

In *A Life's Work*, Rachel Cusk writes of mothers and their children: 'When she is with them, she is not herself; when she is without them, she is not herself; and so it is as difficult to leave your children as it is to stay with them. To discover this is to feel that your life has become irretrievably mired in conflict, or caught in some mythic snare in which you will perpetually, vainly struggle.'

It is comforting to know that my feelings are felt by many mothers. But if new motherhood is hard without fielding a genetic condition, how am I supposed to cope with one? Where's the book about that?

There is also some relief at having a name for Vida's illness, but it comes with fresh worry about what we now have to do. We are dealing with something serious and long-term.

The practical aspects to her care are manifold – and, at this point, I don't know the half of it. Three weekly blood tests and transfusions are both a physical commitment and a mental obstacle: accepting that this is how we keep our daughter alive doesn't come easily.

I know anecdotally, from hovering on parent Facebook groups, that there are all sorts of medical checks needed to maintain a child with DBA. Echocardiograms, ultrasounds and skeletal assessments to check for congenital abnormalities.

Regular biopsies to assess how the condition is evolving in her bone marrow, the body's 'blood factory'. MRIs on the liver, to see how treatments are affecting her. And, sometimes, the steroid trial. I decide to avoid reading up more on these things. I also find myself thinking a lot about my responsibility for Vida's emotional welfare, wondering how the condition could affect her self-image. I never want her to feel lesser because of it, always want her to be secure, confident, able to do all the things that a child without DBA would.

Thing is, that attitude, that ableism, begins at home. A mother in mourning about her diagnosis is not a good start. Before I can just be her mum, I need to accept our difference so that it is just a fact to be navigated. I don't know how I begin to do that.

People keep telling me I need to get used to 'the new normal'. And there is truth to this, but it's a phrase that immediately becomes annoying.

Several people tell me about an essay called 'Welcome to Holland' by Emily Kingsley. It uses the metaphor of going on holiday for having a child with a disability. You are all ready to land in Italy but are redirected to Holland. All the expectations you had of Venice have been dashed by your arrival in, let's say, Utrecht. You've had no time to prepare. Suddenly you need different clothes, new guidebooks, to learn a new language, meet people you hadn't imagined you would. You swap pecorino for Edam, pasta for, well, I think, for what?

Meanwhile, all your old mates go to Italy as planned. You're stuck in Holland. Italy, so full of lovely things, was where you'd planned to go. But you learn that Holland has lovely things to offer too, things that Italy can't.

There's a worthwhile lesson here. But it's too trite to be helpful now, and much too soon to look on the bright side.

I'd really like to just take my daughter to Italy.

One of the advantages to diagnosis is the end of watching and waiting. We know that Vida's body isn't making red blood cells, and with that comes the fact of a transfusion every three weeks. In the week leading up to one, her appetite might dwindle slightly but, on the whole, she doesn't become particularly symptomatic. Her haemoglobin is kept high enough for her to thrive and she is able to get on with the business of being a healthy baby. She is changing fast.

Her cheeks are filling out, and her wrists and ankles have rubber-band fat rolls. Her hair continues to grow, not down but forward, that Tintin quiff ever more impressive. She hates being on her tummy but loves supported standing, pushing her little feet into our laps and smiling with glee. Lots of things interest her, mostly things that aren't toys – remotes, phones, jewellery – and she stares determinedly at an object before going for the grab.

I'm having fun dressing her, too. It has replaced any kind of pleasure I once took in dressing myself. Louise and I make pilgrimages to a children's charity shop in Camden for sartorial treasures. We find a dress covered in pictures of sweet peas for our sweet pea. She has several kimonos, two pairs of sunglasses, a gilet and a Fiorucci T-shirt, and she rocks a bloomer. And, in preparation for autumn, her burgeoning knitwear collection is *par excellence*. Getting Vida dressed in the morning gives me structure, an essential task after changing and feeding her. The necessity of these tasks keeps me going. I also recognise that clothes are a defence. Not only can she have DBA and look like other babies, she can have it and look fucking fabulous.

I'm doing things that I never thought I would when I became a mum. To get her to sleep longer, I am training her to take a bottle of formula every night (although she makes her preference for breastfeeding abundantly clear). I'm also encouraging TV – even at the tender age of five months she watches *Peppa Pig* with wonder. I recognise how valuable it will become on transfusion days, when keeping still is the name of the game.

I'm also heavily reliant on her buggy. I gave up trying to settle her in the cot as soon as we knew she was ill. She didn't like being put down and it caused her distress, making nap times an ordeal for all of us. Much better to get her to nap while she feeds or when we're on the move. She likes the motion of the pram and I start going out for long walks to send her asleep. We rack up quite the step count, covering much of north-west London – Kilburn, Camden High Street, St John's Wood. Most of all, over the Finchley Road, through Frognal and into Hampstead – winding through Church Row, Flask Walk, Well Walk, and onto the heath with its birdsong and fan-like canopy, which shelters us from the sun. I've read online that DBA patients need extra sun protection due to their elevated risk of skin cancer. The shade suits my mood, too. Walking on the heath becomes a kind of therapy, a place where the heat and high spirits of the summer feel less oppressive.

Branches and horse-chestnut leaves shield Vida and me like outstretched palms.

I have very little sense of community during these summer months and spend a lot of the daytimes with Vida only. I am heavy with my thoughts and hate being alone with them, but making conversation with other people can be equally isolating. I identify so much with C. S. Lewis's observation in *A Grief Observed* that, 'There is a sort of invisible blanket between the world and me. I find it hard to take in what anyone says. Or perhaps, hard to want to take it in. It is so uninteresting. Yet I want others to be about me.' I realise that what I'm feeling is grief, and that we can grieve ideas as well as people.

But Vida is very much here. Freddie describes her as 'full of life, but not haemoglobin'. He's right, of course. And so, alongside my constant worry about her, my love for her has grown boundless. It is bigger, even, than her hair.

The word 'normal' keeps coming up. It's the most everyday – normal, you might say – of words, and it's volleyed around all the time, by everyone. Its meaning seems so anodyne; it is a throwaway adjective; certainly, nobody means to cause hurt with it. But I find it piercing. Normal is a word which cuts, its letters are lined with razors. And I am newly aware of how often it is used.

From the start of a child's life, the idea of 'normal' is an unspecific benchmark for development. I accept that Vida's haemoglobin production is not in the 'normal' range, but does this really make her an 'abnormal' child? I push back against the lazy comparisons between her and 'normal' babies made by others, from health visitors and GPs to friends. These occur more than you might think.

What does 'normal' even mean? Surely it's subjective? Used in the context of children who are unwell, it dances around the uncomfortable fact of them being in peril, othering them rather than accepting and celebrating them.

I keep being told to feel grateful that Vida seems so normal. And I *do* feel relief that her condition is invisible – I think it will make life easier for her. I realise I might not feel this way if we lived in a culture that better enabled those with conspicuous differences, and that I have picked up society's attitude to sick children: I am part of the problem. I feel now, at the time of writing, that this conditioning was a major factor in my response to Vida's diagnosis.

There is a lot of emphasis on diversity in the media now and there are programmes, such as *The Baby Club*, that do a good job of representing children from myriad backgrounds. But now that I have a child with 'additional needs', I'm aware of how much work remains to be done. In *Peppa Pig*, for instance, Pedro Pony goes to hospital because he has broken his leg, which is put in plaster and heals. But what about the kids for whom hospital isn't a question of getting fixed or cured? Are their stories too frightening to tell – and so not worth telling?

It's not just important for children like Vida to see their experiences mirrored back to them. It's important for their caregivers, too. Whether it's children's TV or the weekend papers, our otherness, as parents of a seriously ill child, is constantly reinforced by a very narrow take on what is normal.

People keep telling Freddie and me that we're being so strong, that we're doing a great job. These are kindnesses, but they also mark out our difference. I know that as a mother I *am* normal. The sheer fact of having a child with a condition does not make me an extraordinary parent. Nor does educating myself about the disease, finding her the best care, or holding her still while yet another needle is put into her elbow. What other choice do I have? Wouldn't everyone do the same? This is a normal, ordinary mother's love.

Hospitals do, of course, feature in lots of children's books and television. It's not just Pedro Pony who goes to hospital and gets fixed; Maisy Mouse does, too, after she falls off her trampoline, and in Julia Donaldson's wonderful story *Hospital Dog* – about a Dalmatian who works as a therapy dog on a paediatric ward – children's colds are cleared, temperatures are brought down, fractures healed.

The message is almost always that hospitals make you better. Such was the cushioning I had received. My thirty-four years have been unscathed by the serious threat of illness to anyone close to me. There were admissions to hospital – my dad had two heart attacks, and my mum, who is asthmatic, had a nasty brush with pneumonia when I was about ten and spent several weeks in hospital. But they both came home better. Medicine mended.

Early on in all this, I'd had a blind faith that whatever was causing Vida's anaemia would be sorted out by the hospital. Now that we have a diagnosis, I feel a bit cheated – by medicine, which can only help us to manage Vida's condition, and by the naivety that had cosseted me. I feel perverse resentment about having been so fortunate up until now. I have had absolutely no training for this: no warm-up for emergency healthcare, let alone caring for a child with a chronic illness.

I crave something that might help me with my feelings of otherness, but I'm not sure what. Certainly, it feels too soon to talk. Therapy requires reflection, friendships require dialogue. I need something private, one-sided, my own. It's not as easy as you might imagine to find things to read. There are the testimonies of other parents on charity websites like Genetic Disorders UK, and some DBA families have spoken to the press, but this kind of material taps into my fear of DBA overwhelming our family life. I need somehow to acknowledge the hugeness of what we face without letting it feel bigger than me. What I want are the stories of people who have absorbed their child's diagnosis into their everyday; I need to be able to hope that something of the person I was for three and a half decades before motherhood can remain. Even better, I want to read the stories of parents who seem bolstered by these challenges.

I imagine a time in the future when I might write the thing I feel to be missing, but quickly forget about it. Few things have ever seemed so impossible.

Now that I am on the receiving end of people's condolences, I think about how I must have got it wrong in the past. I had been a dealer in glibness and now find those trite encouragements of mine – 'stay strong', 'be positive', 'keep calm' – echoed back to me by orbiting sympathisers. The blind faith of others is alienating, when what I want, or need, from them is to be joined at the front line of my fear. I also hear a lot of 'I don't know how you do it' and 'I can't even imagine', to which I always want to say, 'Well, why don't you try?'

It makes me think of 'Oh Dearism', a phrase coined by the filmmaker Adam Curtis to describe how Western audiences respond to television news, which often presents them with horrifying scenes of human suffering. We feel powerless to do anything to help, so we say 'oh dear' and put what we have seen in a compartment labelled 'Difficult' in our mental filing cabinet. Is that what Freddie and I have become to our friends? I imagine people exchanging grimaces and saying 'poor them' over swaying glasses of wine at parties before moving onto the subject of holiday plans.

In kinder, more reasonable moments, I wonder what the hell people *should* say? Even 'I'm so sorry', which *does* meet me where I am, feels problematic: no one should apologise for Vida. This is, of course, not what people mean to imply when they tell me they are sorry, but language is thorny territory. I am forever caught in its brambles. In *Notes on Grief*, Chimamanda Ngozi Adichie hits the nail on the head: 'Grief is about language, the failure of language and the grasping for language.'

As well as the line about adapting to the 'new normal', I'm also hearing the likes of 'it's what Vida will know' and 'she won't know any different'. This is true and, in later months, it will offer a rational prism through which to view the life experience my daughter will have. But in these early months, it's an idea that overlooks the simple fact that I don't want it to be all she will know. I don't want her childhood punctuated – or punctured? – by needles. When people philosophise in this way, it jumps ahead, skips my grief. I need time to be sad.

Many people are worried about Vida and what her diagnosis will mean for her (not least because typing 'Diamond-Blackfan anaemia' into a search engine paints a bleak and outdated picture). I appreciate them taking the time to research, also to ask questions, see clearly what we are facing. But I also can't be responsible for allaying their fears when I already have so many of my own. It is quite enough to manage the needs of a baby alongside my feelings.

Words, then, have become fearsome, exiling. I become selective not just about what I read, but who I see and speak to.

'We have happy memories, even before transplant,' says the woman's voice over the phone. I believe her and find myself hanging onto her words. Whenever I feel this way about someone, be they Freddie, a doctor or, in this case, a stranger, I worry instantly about the conversation's end – their final sentence, the full stop, the goodbye – which leaves me alone with DBA again. I can feel hopeful, but only under supervision; I have no self-sufficiency in this arena. I need regular transfusions of donor positivity.

In my googling, I have fallen upon a blog written in 2008 by the parents of a child with DBA, who was at the time having a bone-marrow transplant. The family's journey to this point was eventful; after three rounds of IVF with PGD they had a matched child, a potential donor for their sibling. The mother, who I'm speaking to now, is also a journalist; this, combined with her clearly unstoppable approach and her manner – which avoids sugar-coating 'hideous' DBA but offers a bright outlook (the transplant was successful) – draws me to her. I trust her. I want to do this her way.

She is one of a handful of DBA elders I meet over the summer. I leech onto their pragmatism and I appreciate their kindness when they say things like, 'Vida will be OK because she has you. We just have to make sure that *you're* OK.' Other people have said things like this to me too, but the elders are walking, talking survivors, proof that there is life beyond the DBA echo chamber I'm currently living in.

Around the same time, once Vida is officially diagnosed, I speak to Al Gilmour's wife, Emily. They are in the thick of their son's steroid trial, a period spent behind closed doors with a supercharged, often angry, sometimes sleepless toddler. The summer is a goldfish bowl for Emily and me: we look out on the world enjoying itself. Emily is matter-of-fact about how difficult she finds it, also uncomplaining. Why can't I just get on with it like her?

Emily and every other mother is emphatic: go and see Dr Josu de la Fuente. I get the ball rolling on this and ask Dr Alamelu to make the referral to him – she was once his registrar.

Let's hope Dr Jesus lives up to his name. And Vida to hers.

A family outing! It is mid-July and we have our first appointment with Dr Josu at St Mary's Hospital in Paddington. My parents have made the journey from south London, and we from West Hampstead. It took all of fifteen minutes to get here: one DBA specialist in the country and he's based down the road. In time, this will feel convenient, but at this moment there is an eeriness to having spent so much of my life just a stone's throw from a place so vital to my daughter's wellbeing. A parallel life awaited me a mere postcode away.

Despite the hospital's proximity, we are running late. I jump out of the car at Regent's Canal, just behind the hospital, and head inside while the others look for parking. Surprisingly, for a place where prime ministers and royalty have had their babies, St Mary's feels in need of some love – peeling paint, halogen-lit, not enough windows. Not all hospitals are created equal, and the Evelina has set the bar high.

I sit in a waiting area; a unicorn grins at me on the wall. Nurses go in and out of a small room, loading up trays with bottles and sterile packets of things from little drawers: the apparatus for cannulation, a phlebotomy buffet. I see an energetic toddler go into the room with his mum, who smiles and exchanges a pleasantry with one of the nurses. I can only assume the boy has had a bone-marrow transplant – his face is puffy on steroids, spiky tufts of soft hair emerge from his scalp. I find the mother's cheeriness brave and unfathomable. How does she do it? Living in the moment, as illness often requires, is a tall order for parents. We fear always what we might lose.

It's a hot day and the unit seems airless. It doesn't help that I can't breathe through my nose for, briefly alone, I am safe to cry. I've lost any shame about doing so in front of strangers. A nurse with dark hair approaches and introduces herself as the DBA clinical nurse specialist. She asks if I'm Vida's mum, and when I confirm that I am, every duct on my face releases itself. 'Grotesque, without solution,' as Lorca wrote of weeping. I throb with fresh grief, cry hot tears. In my own and other people's flushed ears, veiny hands, mottled legs, I am reminded of the genius of our bodies, producing 2 million red blood cells every minute without even knowing it.

'It's a lot,' the nurse says softly. She sits with me quietly until the others arrive. I plough through a box of tissues and leave a cup of water untouched. We are ushered into the clinic room and meet Josu, sitting on a swivel chair in a three-piece suit. He warmly remarks on how much support we have, with all three grandparents in tow, and coos at Vida, who I can tell is not going to sit through this. She seems to have inherited my fear of missing out – and while FOMO might be the least of my worries these days, at five months old Vida has many better places to be than a small room in a hospital with seven adults talking in risk statistics, timeframes, numbers.

And numbers there are. Today is perhaps a new low for me; in spite of Josu's jolly demeanour, the information he delivers – some of it familiar from my reading, some of it new – is hard to hear.

Vida's DBA is a classic case, he says: she is in the 60 per cent who present in their first twelve weeks. Her haemoglobin level on admission was extremely low, as were the reticulocytes (young red blood cells), which her bone marrow should have been producing to make up for the severe anaemia. These were the clangers, the emergency symptoms, but there are lots of other indicators, he says, 'which are always remarkably easy to see in retrospect'. The high Doppler reading before she was born ('lots of women have that'); her slightly raised foetal haemoglobin; her heart murmur, which is common to many newborns; her elevated eADA protein (not enough to prove a diagnosis on its own).

He clearly has a spiel that he must give. There is no good way to deliver headlines like these. When Vida turns one, she will start a course of high-dose steroids. Steroids are the lightest intervention, but for plenty of patients they don't work, or they stop working. She has an 80 per cent chance of responding to them, but only a minority of patients can maintain their response at a dose that isn't harmful. For now, the only treatment that we can rely on is transfusions.

Life on transfusions is a balancing act: untreated bone-marrow failure is incompatible with life, yet, if used long-term, the transfusions used to treat it can be too. Iron overload is a serious concern. To offset it, there is chelation, but this can then play havoc with the liver, kidneys, sight and hearing. It's a multidisciplinary tightrope walk, and we are looking at many days in hospital for the foreseeable future. In Vida's first eighteen months, she will have some twenty blood transfusions, but also appointments with specialists to address possible issues with her heart, kidneys, immune system, gut and liver.

Also starting after her first birthday will be periodic biopsies to check the health of Vida's bone marrow. He tells us that a small proportion of patients will have a spontaneous remission for an unknown period of time. As if by magic, their bone marrow starts to produce a healthy number of red cells. But this luck can also reverse at any time. I tell Josu that I don't want Vida to be shackled to hospitals her whole life. 'A lot of children do very well on them,' he says, and tells us about some of the highly successful adults in this care – 'You'd never know.'

I make it known that I have done some research, that despite my appearance, I am ready to battle this thing and get Vida the bone marrow transplant that will liberate her from life on transfusions and chelation. He emphasises a transplant's risks, that it is a treatment usually reserved for children who have exhausted other things, or who have a sibling match – because it has historically been considered safer than with an unrelated donor. I tell him that I've been looking into IVF. We want more children anyway, I say, so trying to have one who is a match makes sense.

Freddie and I might not yet be sure if we want Vida to have a transplant, but the idea of her not having to come to hospital every three weeks, or the side effects from transfusions, is compelling. I'm aware that the decision to do it would be massive, that the process is far from straightforward. I also know that transplants are controversial in the DBA community, no two ever the same, full of variables that are impossible to predict. But in this first meeting, I am communicating something else: I want everyone here to know that I am ready. That I still have my fight.

Josu both indulges and reins me in. He goes along with my plan, agreeing to refer us for IVF with pre-implantation genetic diagnosis, meanwhile suggesting I focus on enjoying this beautiful baby – who is currently shrieking with boredom outside in the corridor with Louise.

—

It strikes me that the doctors we have met since all this began have seen a rawer, perhaps truer, version of me than my friends possibly ever have. They've witnessed my nature at its most elemental, unbound by pleasantries – my fury, my fire; my self-assurance, arrogance even, when I ask questions; my swiftness to act, my impatience; the dynamics with my family members; my bullishness alongside the measured quietness of my husband. Until now I have deployed a cordial glaze; new acquaintances might have described me with adjectives like 'lovely', 'sweet', 'nice' – I realised early on that female ambition is most palatable in vanilla flavour – my true nature hidden from plain sight. By those standards, today has been grossly self-exposing. And while I am aware of that, I don't feel self-conscious or embarrassed. I wonder if this is one of only a few acceptable scenarios for a woman to show her mettle so unapologetically? As mothers, we can be fierce in ways that I doubt would wash in other contexts. I leave the consultation tingling with catharsis, from having the appointment I'd been waiting weeks for, but also from displaying myself unhindered by a lifetime's learnt behaviour.

It is obvious to me that, for all the suboptimality of DBA's treatments, we are very lucky to be facing a Diamond-Blackfan diagnosis in 2019, after the arrival of iron chelation in particular. Likewise, we are fortunate that London is our home, where the country's only specialist in this nuanced – and, frankly, baffling – condition is based, and where we have our pick of world-famous children's hospitals to help us monitor Vida's multifaceted medical needs.

What no decade, city or hospital can offer us, though, is certainty about how this is all going to play out.

People love to tell me that none of us can be certain of what awaits us. We can't, and in this respect, yes, maybe Vida is typical of the human condition. But this is also too simplistic; let's not pretend that the task of parents with unwell children is the same as for those whose kids are healthy. In a society in which having a sick child is everyone's worst fear, where is the precedent for finding peace in our situation? How will I enjoy the mundane delights of motherhood – first words, first steps, first dunk of a chip in ketchup – when always there lurks the possibility of my worst fear?

Vida and I take the train down to Streatham, where Mum has made lunch. I anticipate seeing her with a mixture of relief and trepidation. Walking through my parents' front door, some of my tension uncoils as I am hit by the smells of home: quiche, dark wood furniture, a hoover full of dog hair. Frank, our elderly Staffie, waddles up to me, wagging his tail with his whole body and grunting; I'm sure he knows I'm not doing well – whenever I'm here, he sits loyally at my feet, looks for my hand and roots at the edge of it so I stroke his crown. I like Frank's style of support. I'm heavily reliant on Mum and Dad's support too, but also irritated by their efforts to be positive.

Today, Mum has asked her friend Liz over. Liz was Mum's mentor when she did NCT during her pregnancy with me. The two lived opposite one another on an ungentrified south-

London street in the mid-1980s, and Liz's daughter Ellie – my oldest friend, now senior in NHS management, no less – was born eighteen months prior to me. While ours was a home run by two journalists for whom good stories were everything, grey areas celebrated and multiple truths possible, Liz and Paul have all the clear-sighted pragmatism of mathematicians. They came at things from another angle to my parents, and in this difference there was magnetism. When I arrive in Streatham to find Liz there, I know what Mum is hoping for – a rhetoric that might help me see some light.

I can feel everyone's fatigue. DBA, its treatments, and IVF are all I talk about. Sometimes other people engage and my fire is stoked by words spoken out loud, as though these conversations make the possibility of Vida becoming transfusion-independent more real. Other times, they are tired of it and try to distract me: Freddie with meal-planning, Mum with offers to have Vida so I can read or get a haircut, or even think about a keeping-in-touch day at work. All of this seems so decadent. Work! I hadn't known true work before now. And leisure! Films or books or any kind of extra-curricular activity strike me not only as frippery, but dangerous. Whenever we watch TV together, or buy a sandwich up the road, or walk the dog, I see only people with bone marrow that, I assume, works. Other people's apparent health is everywhere to wallop me. There is no escape from it.

Freddie has recently reminded me, pointedly, that Vida is the one with the condition, not me. He's right. Where is my selfless maternal stoicism, a quality that my own mother has in spades? I have taken this diagnosis badly, I know, a fact that is laced with guilt for me.

'I wanted to talk to you,' says Liz, pulling up a chair at the kitchen table as Mum hovers in the background, bobbing up and down with Vida in her arms.

I am trying not to cry. I have known this woman my whole life, probably cried in front of her dozens of times as a child, but I seldom see her these days and I am suddenly aware of my shame. Shame at the lump in my throat, the rising sting in my face, the quiver in my lip; also shame at her having reason to talk to me in this way at all. This is new terrain for us – adult to adult, I no longer a child in her care. The dynamic has shifted now, and her message is simple: this might be hard, but I have a responsibility to Vida.

The more I try to hold it together, the more inevitable crying becomes. I give in, sinking my upper body – with its knotted muscles, sorrow held in each sinew – onto the kitchen table.

Liz reminds me that I can't fall apart, that Vida is going to need a lot of support over the course of her life and that I have to be strong for her. She delivers this gently but firmly. I daren't answer back, as I would if she were my mum. Petulance zipped in, I am forced to hear what I know is expected of me, the things that, said out loud, scare me so much. That I am an advocate for my daughter, no matter her treatment pathway; that I have a duty not only to educate myself about this condition, but to fight for her wellbeing at every juncture.

In her Neapolitan novels, Elena Ferrante writes about the character Lila's 'dissolving margins'. I had inhaled these books a few years back, but perhaps never known what she'd meant with this phrase until now. The pressure to be a good mother makes me feel as though I am melting; I can't contain this sea of worry within the framework of myself. I am all liquid. Perverse as it is, I can summon the energy to push for the most extreme approach to treating Diamond-Blackfan – to make a sibling donor so my daughter can have a bone-marrow transplant and be haematologically (if not genetically) cured – but all the miniature degrees between here and there feel like a bigger feat. The always questioning of clinicians; pushing to make her every brush with hospital comfortable and safe; the staying abreast of research; most importantly, to imbue her with a sense of her own magnificence, both in spite of and because of her medical challenges. For her always to feel like she is everything I want her to be and more, the only version of Vida that the world needs.

'I just don't think I can do it, Liz,' I whisper.

'But she's *here* . . .' she says, her eyes full as she gestures to Vida. Mum's gaze is averted downwards, her lips pursed. I feel bounced into this conversation, at once wildly angry about it and grateful that the issue is being forced through a medium like Liz's tough love. 'And you're already doing it,' she adds.

It's not the first time someone has said this to me. The expectation to put my child's wellbeing above my own can feel oppressive, but while I push against it, I also know that it's what I do anyway. In this way, I have become split, reserving my anger for my mother – she, I think, has no idea what this is like, having had two healthy babies – while going through the motions of looking after and loving Vida unconditionally.

She is taking a bottle at bedtime more happily now and drinks a good bellyful while we read books to her – among them, *Mr Crum's Potato Predicament*, about the invention of potato chips, and *Goodnight Moon*, a weird American classic set in a large bedroom with an old rabbit lady in a rocking chair and her various possessions. These books will be the foundations on which her first words are built, a year or so from now.

Vida's blood tests, transfusions and medical appointments have, for now, joined the other routine logistics of having a baby – nappy changes, feeds, bathtimes. Liz is right, I am already doing it. I am, as I've seen people say on Facebook, 'a DBA mum'.

Whenever we get home after a transfusion, I take a selfie of Vida on my lap, her little cheeks ruddy, her ears glowing and her lips bud-like once more. I, too, look less sallow, revived by the fact of her feeling well. I shared my blood supply with this baby for nine months and now, it seems, she shares hers with me.

For my twenty-first birthday, my cousin Katharine had my birth chart drawn up. I had always wanted it done and hoped that, in plotting the coordinates of my birthday – the time, date, year and the planets' positioning as I sprang from my mother's loins – I would receive a personalised forecast of all the sunny spells that awaited me in life.

Many years on and I remember very little of its contents, except for the section about family. 'You will have a child who is dyslexic or deaf,' it said. I read and reread this sentence, looking for any loopholes in the premonition, or reasons to doubt its truth.

In the days that followed, I was unable to forget it. I was unsettled by the idea of such specific predetermination. Also by the disparity between dyslexia and deafness; as my aunt

Mary said, 'Did the astrologer just look up and see a big D in the sky?'

Dismissing it as hocus pocus, my mum ultimately confiscated the birth chart, only for it to be rediscovered during a loft clear-out not long after her first grandchild was diagnosed with Diamond-Blackfan anaemia.

Of course it was all a coincidence, but I'd be lying if I said it didn't play on my mind sometimes, like the sight of a lone magpie at the beginning of a bad day.

On the day we received Vida's diagnosis, Freddie and I had blood tests to see if either of us carried the mutation, a tiny deletion on a gene called RPS19, which we know to be the one which most commonly causes Diamond-Blackfan. While neither Freddie nor I had ever had issues with our bone marrow, one of us could have dormant DBA and passed it on to Vida, as well as any future children.

We are both negative. There is still a small chance that one of us carries the condition in our reproductive cells – known as mosaicism – although we are told it is more likely to have been a spontaneous occurrence. The chances of her having DBA at all were tiny, unplottable on a graph, the slimmest of slivers on a pie chart. Once again, I ask myself over and over, how and why did this happen?

I abandoned science when, aged sixteen, I realised that I was probably too squeamish to realise my dream of being a vet: during a week of work experience, I fainted while a cat was being neutered. That day changed the course of life for both the cat and myself. I went back to school after the holidays, changed all my A-levels to arts subjects and promised myself I'd always have a dog. Now, however, I need science once more.

I have tracked down a geneticist at St George's, a straight-talking clinician who speaks to me not just as a patient's parent but as the mother of a vulnerable child whose future has been redirected into lonely territory. I warm to her instantly.

She tells me that every human being has roughly sixty new mutations which are not inherited from their parents. Most of the time these mutations are harmless, so you'd have no idea that they even exist. But in Vida's case, the minute deletion on the gene RPS19 has invisible but severe implications. I tell her that I feel we have failed our daughter by giving her faulty DNA. The thing is, she says, without the mutation, Vida wouldn't be the daughter I have. She'd be a different child, born of a different sperm or egg. Vida cannot be Vida without it. This gives me pause. While DBA is essential to Vida on paper, it is as significant to *who* she is as we make it.

The geneticist tells me that there is currently a study taking place at Oxford, a piece of research which could shed light on Freddie's and my specific risk of recurrence as the parents of a child with a *de novo* condition. I leap at this. Whether or not we end up having another child using IVF, it would help to know for sure, not just to suspect, that the chances of DBA happening again are low. She makes the referral.

In August, Mum and I take Vida to Norfolk, where my parents have a small cottage. This place is something like a family headquarters for us; our roots run deep here. My mother's side has farmed in the area for generations, and my paternal grandparents moved here in the 1950s, seduced by the sea and a house that looked out over it. In the seventies, my parents met in Norwich, both trainees on the *Eastern Daily Press*. Freddie and I also met in Norfolk; his stepmother and siblings live just up the road.

I grew up in London but Norfolk is a home of sorts, always there for high days, holidays, and the days I wanted to end: break-ups, schoolgirl squabbles, brief sadnesses I couldn't put a name to, all of them called for Norfolk, my salty tonic. More than love the place, which I do – the North Sea with its crunch of ancient shingle; the summer's sweeps of wheat and, later, bales, like sausage rolls on the flat horizon; the River Glaven and the ford, where I and my parents and their parents before them have thrown stones for the dog and played Pooh sticks – I feel it bound up in my body, a genetic tie that is as much a part of me as the mole on my nose or my small, always rather wrinkled hands.

When I became pregnant, I'd imagined spending chunks of my maternity leave in Norfolk. I wanted our daughter to know this place deep in her bones, too – for it to be as much an extension of her as it had been for me. What I hadn't imagined was today's scenario, Mum and I driving up the M11 with a full car and screaming baby. In Thetford Forest, we pull over so I can feed. Mum leans over and massages my head, pressing her fingertips into my unwashed scalp. She so wants to make this nice, to relieve me. I wish she could. I wonder if she feels as helpless about my suffering as I do about Vida's, then reel at the awfulness of parenthood. A confluence of extreme love, anguish and responsibility – it is too much to bear. I wish she had warned me.

By the time we arrive, it's a beautiful afternoon. Mum spreads a rug out in the garden and we lie the baby on it in the shade. The grass is strewn with daisies and I absently make Vida a chain, which I dangle above her. She goes cross-eyed, makes a grab for it. Mum brings me tea – a perfect raw umber; how is it that nobody can make a cup of tea like my mum? – and we pick at a polenta cake that has defrosted en route, a trans-county bake. It is not exactly how I'd imagined spending time in Norfolk on maternity leave, and the tightness in my chest is always there, but the change of scenery feels good. I see how Vida is noticing the new environment. She is lulled by the country noises: branches shaken by breeze, the calls of a wood pigeon, the odd moo from the meadow.

During this week, I have a little repose with a roster of granny and step-granny and great-aunt at the ready to whisk Vida down the lane in the pram for a sleep while I sit in the stillness of the garden. In the old days I filled empty time with reading or cooking or drinks, lots of drinks. Now, when I am briefly without my baby, I adjust to the tingle of her absence, and pause.

Sometimes it seems as though I am living my life in negative, like a roll of film. Before, there had been the odd shadow to an otherwise mostly light existence. Now, I live in a lot of shade, gloomy days lit up by my baby's smile and small victories like my conversation with the geneticist. She had started a rationalising process in me. She'd likened Vida's mutation to a spelling mistake that has fundamentally changed the meaning of a sentence:

'The cause is not known.'

But what if this had been mistyped?

'The cause is now known.'

Here, the change of a single letter not only reads well – all five words are still legitimate and the sentence is grammatical – but the meaning of the clause is fundamentally changed. If I had been proofreading an article and missed this error, it would have been a significant oversight: its meaning is qualitatively different from that of the intended sentence. This, more than one geneticist tells me, is similar to what happens when people have small but serious mutations like Vida's. Her system reads her genetic code and gets the wrong idea.

We sign up to the study that the geneticist had told me about, called PREGCARE, and I start to look into the nuts and bolts of IVF. I feel great compassion for anyone who has had to have a child this way; the stress levels are as high as the stakes. We have always wanted more than one child, and we agree that if there's a way of having one who could someday help their sister, we should explore it. Freddie is reluctant to think about another baby while I am so unstable (he doesn't use that word, but I know that's what he means). For several months he has lived with someone unable to keep a steady perspective on things, someone in need of regular reassurance. As well as getting my ducks in a row for IVF, I need to convince Freddie that I can keep them there.

I feel increasingly stable in my determination to make this happen; I have a sense of being able to shape things for Vida and this fuels me. I gather written confirmation of her mutation and a formal referral from our genetics team so that an application can be made to the Human Fertilisation and Embryology Authority (HFEA), and I look into IVF clinics.

I take to all of this feverishly, like an assignment with a deadline of yesterday. I work hard, aware that this is quite literally my life's work. I march around London with the buggy and, while Vida sleeps, I make calls and write emails, gathering the information I need to advance our plot – a plot I'm determined to have some control over.

My progress is both exhausting and energising. Amid it all, and Vida's hospital appointments, however, there's also the regular stuff: bottles; broken sleep; immunisations; her first temperature. In some ways these things are the hardest. A mother has to be so many people. Chronic illness just reveals another dimension of the role.

It's also a role that evolves with my daughter. My skills now extend to entertainer and tour guide – singing songs, pulling faces, and offering her objects to inspect. She is ready for her world to expand and I am her gateway.

Bedtime remains tricky. She will fall asleep in my arms, either feeding against the undulations of my breath, or bouncing on the birthing ball, which is giving me a bad back. When I put her down in her cot, she'll often cry out and the process will begin all over again. I crave a child-free evening, just an hour to myself. When I eventually get downstairs to Freddie and Louise, we'll breathe a sigh of relief, then see out the day watching videos of Vida on my phone.

I wonder if there's a word for this. For needing a break from someone, but not being able to get enough of them. I suppose it's motherhood.

—

We have been sent a box of collection materials by the people from the PREGCARE study at Oxford University, vials for samples of our various body fluids: urine, saliva, semen and mouth swabs. We are instructed to fill these up and bring them with us to St George's in Tooting. We schlep down on a sweaty Northern line and a researcher takes blood from us. The materials collected, they are sent off and forgotten about. It won't be until the following spring that we get the results, indicating where Vida's mutation came from. It will tell us that neither Fred nor I have DBA in any of our cells, meaning for definite that Vida's was indeed a completely random event and that the chances of her having DBA were infinitesimal.

Professor Andrew Wilkie is one of two clinical geneticists at Oxford who led the study. When we speak to discuss our results, I find out he has children of his own. And this prompts me to ask him what I have been wondering: how anyone with his knowledge of all the things that can go awry in the production of a human can go on to produce a human of their own without going insane in the process.

'Our knowledge of blood is wide yet unfinished,' wrote Rose George in her brilliant book *Nine Pints*. This is what I keep coming up against. I am as incredulous about everything that is known about my daughter's blood condition as I am about everything that isn't. Even the world's greatest experts on DBA can't answer some of my questions. Genetic code and bone marrow conspire in obscure ways to produce a condition that baffles great medical minds. The general consensus, though, is that blood production is the most demanding process our bodies perform. ('We don't entirely know why DBA presents in the blood, or why it is mostly a red-cell issue, but we do know that we make more blood cells than anything else,' Josu told me.)

Prof Wilkie's team has sequenced Vida's genome and matched it up to the UCSC Genome Browser. It shows her mutation on RPS19 and compares the *correct* sequencing of RPS19 in human beings to a host of apes, a bushbaby, a mouse and a dog. They are all identical at this particular position; all mammalian species have exactly the same sequence in their RPS19 gene, which, as Prof Wilkie says 'is a measure of the fact that this is a very important protein doing very important things. Evolution hasn't allowed it to vary at all.'

These science lessons from doctors help me because it makes things feel less personal: we are subject to the same natural variation as all living things. Moreover, until this point, acquiring information about DBA has felt frightening. Now I get my first flavour of knowledge as power.

But what is power exactly, in a situation like this, where the diagnosis is so serious? At the beginning, I had imagined that Vida would be brought back to health with a transfusion and a week's stay at our local hospital. With her diagnosis came the realisation that we were not in a position to cure, only to manage. And as long as I craved a cure, wished for her not to have DBA, felt guilty and sad that she did, I could only ever feel defeat. With a new understanding of the boundaries – that my daughter has this illness, that this gene mutation is the reason, that there are things we can do and things we can't – I reason that we can protect her in the ways that science knows.

We got good news from the PREGCARE study: our risk of recurrence is low, almost nil. But I don't think it was just the results that helped things to take a turn for me – it was new understanding. I had struggled profoundly with the unknown cause of Vida's DBA, but after an explanation from geneticists, it feels less like a cosmic conspiracy.

Institutional decor is familiar now, mostly at doctors' surgeries or hospital clinics. Their wipe-clean surfaces create echoes that support my general sense of gloom. But this department of a central London hospital is different. Here there are soft furnishings, padded chairs with angles that aren't quite comfortable, scratchy carpets, tissue boxes on every tabletop or counter. I sip water from a polystyrene cup, fill in some multiple-choice questions on a clipboard, a pen attached to it with tape and string.

I am here for my first cognitive behavioural therapy (CBT) session. This hospital is geographically close to my office, yet feels light years away. I don't feel optimistic about what CBT will offer me but, in the spirit of showing willingness to help myself, here I am. Mum has been pushing for me to see what mental health support is available on the NHS. Sitting here is the upshot of a long effort involving various phone consultations, e-surveys and form filling. In fact, I'm sure I've filled in this particular form before. From a selection of answers, it asks me how frequently I've felt things like pleasure, shame, hopelessness or suicidal ideation recently.

There's a grim comedy to it all that feels singularly British to me. It has a whiff of Mike Leigh – the place and its personnel are of a type, and I experience them through a dimly lit lens of 1980s filmmaking. Onscreen they'd be parody; here they are flatly unironic.

A bearded therapist – about my age, wearing turned-up trousers and thick-rimmed glasses – peers out from a room, looks at his own clipboard, pauses. 'Ex-im . . . Ssshhmina . . .?'

'Mina,' I say, helping him out. I've had thirty-four years of official types (teachers, doctors, now therapists) not being able to pronounce my Spanish name, Ximena. A shortening has always been essential.

It's late afternoon on a wet autumn day, a mirror to my mood. The therapist invites me into a consulting room with blinds to cover a glass wall overlooking the corridor; he closes them with a toggle, sits down and crosses his leg, which hitches up a trouser leg to reveal plimsolls I might once have admired. Not long ago I enjoyed putting outfits together; now I might see something in a shop window, feel tempted, then remember that I can't like anything. Involuntarily, multiple times a day, I censor my thoughts in this way.

'So, Mina, how have you been feeling?'

I tell him what has happened, summarising: 'I feel a lot of grief and a sense of hopelessness.'

He cocks his head, purses his lips, nods. 'Hmm, OK ... sounds like you're feeling some grief and hopelessness.'

'Yes.'

'And what do you think the triggers might be for feeling this way?'

I explain that I find it difficult to hear about other people's experiences of having children. Their 'normal' worries and priorities, like childcare and routines, all of it seems so close but like such a dream.

'Hmm, yeah, that makes sense.' He pauses, writes something on his clipboard.

As many first sessions do, the appointment becomes about context – me giving the therapist the background, telling him what we've been through in recent months – the terrifyingly low blood count, the transfusions, the unknown future.

Towards the end, he looks up, 'Oh, I've been meaning to ask, are you able to meet half an hour earlier in future? It would just be great to be able to get back home in time for my daughter's bath.'

There we go again, I think, alienated by another parent's normal reality. I suppose this is why therapists are often guarded about their personal lives: the sharing of a quotidian fact can be a devastating reveal.

Meanwhile, my mum is pushing the buggy around St Pancras station. Vida is wearing her first winter coat and resembles a powder-pink Michelin man riding in a wheeled throne. Mum's trepidation around me is increasingly evident; I ache at being its cause but feel powerless to stop it.

In the Romantic period, melancholy was looked upon as something to be admired: it made its sufferer interesting, it brought them inspiration, depth. This always resonated with me. Before I had Vida, I enjoyed crunching over my issues with friends and wine. We interrogated our sadnesses, and maybe that did make us more interesting? But I don't feel that way about this. It has emptied me.

CBT sets out to arm the patient with personal coping mechanisms, retraining unhelpful thought processes that may not be serving them. In the past, I'd had limited interest in CBT, preferring to 'go deeper' with a psychotherapist (although I hadn't ever stuck with it long-term because of the cost). But, arguably, in my current state, I don't have the luxury of time.

Which is how I end up sitting opposite the bearded therapist. He is probably a nice guy, but every week he manages to alienate me with his practised compassion and bureaucratic box-ticking. I go to three of these weekly sessions, and before each one I have to complete a survey to help the service measure my progress. But is how I feel quantifiable? And if it is, what kind of timeframe is realistic?

Looking back, it's hard to believe how many therapists I saw in Vida's first year, each time wanting to be saved from myself, unable to comprehend what a long road lay ahead.

The parent counsellor at the Evelina had not heard of DBA. I spent nearly an hour explaining the condition to her through tears. She looked on sympathetically, made helpless 'Ohh' noises when I sobbed, and then I left, dehydrated.

—

The months roll on and even I have to admit that I'm not getting better. One, two, three and four months after Vida's diagnosis, and hope feels like another time zone. I resist antidepressants; 'I'm still breastfeeding,' I say, but I know anecdotally from friends that antidepressants can make things feel worse before they get better. Could things be worse? What is 'better'? I am wary of numbing myself, but maybe numbness would be better than this?

I tell my mum that I don't want to be here anymore. What I mean is that I'd like to disappear, probably just to fall asleep, but she hears something else. In a spin, she pushes for a psychiatric referral, and I meet with a psychiatrist at Guy's Hospital. He is unusually warm for a clinician and handsome, too; even in my state of not-caring, I'm suddenly aware of how unkempt I am. I tell him everything; he makes quiet listening noises. He tells me he could prescribe a course of antidepressants if I want, but that he suspects my depression is in fact a rational response to the circumstances.

For the first time, I really feel someone has understood where I am. Everyone I'd seen until this point had cemented my sense of being sole resident on a small, faraway island for the parents of children with rare illnesses. But the psychiatrist acknowledges the trauma and says, essentially, your reaction is reasonable.

I might be devastated, but I'm not mad.

The grannies have taken a scattergun approach to getting help for me. Recommendations for therapists are rolling in from their friends and contacts. I see another, this time based barely a stone's throw from Louise's house. My mum wheels Vida off for an hour, and once more, I find myself relaying the year so far.

I explain DBA and the tortuous wait for a diagnosis. I am weary of speaking about it and realise that saying it aloud – in 'talking therapy' – isn't doing much to help. I feel as shredded as the damp and disintegrating tissue in my hand. The therapist tells me that she too has a daughter with a genetic disorder. A grown-up, accomplished daughter, with two children of her own, who 'does not want to be taken as less – different, maybe – but will not let her health challenge stop her from doing anything'.

My ears prick up. I wish I could say that, in that moment, I saw in this therapist the makings of the one I'd been looking for, but really, I simply hung onto the words of this older woman – gracious, groomed, successful and, from what I could tell, happy – who'd been through something similar.

And so began an unconventional therapist-patient relationship. I spoke to this therapist every few weeks for about a year and grew to know more about her than was perhaps typical of our arrangement, and when I asked her if this is just her style – do all her patients know these things about her? – she said no, but she saw how isolated I felt on that first day and suspected I would find it useful.

The next time, she asks me to take Vida, and from then on, we see her for therapy together. I don't realise it, but I am not talking to my baby as much as I should. I'm excellent at singing 'Old MacDonald' to calm her cries, but everyday chatter and eye contact make me nervous, a reminder of what I could have lost. The therapist tells me that Vida needs to look into my eyes and see joy, not grief; hope, not despair; can, not can't.

With swatches of textured fabric and wooden blocks, glittery magic wands and brightly coloured feathers, a squidgy knobbly ball and a maraca, I learn the makings of play with my daughter. Propping her up between cushions (she is still prone to toppling over), I look at the wonder in her eyes when she sees something new, and how her chubby little hands reach out to grab, shake or thwack while she chortles.

Since that first session, this therapist and I have discussed often the provision of mental-health services for parents and carers of children with chronic illnesses. There is little that tunes into the fear that parents of newly diagnosed children feel, or that goes with them on the journey they will inevitably have to take.

'It seems that the system of care is more interested in noting differences than in welcoming them,' she says. 'After that, healthcare professionals tend to leave patients and their parents to it, rather than accompanying them.' Vida's medical care is some of the best in the world, but what about Freddie and me? We may not have the condition, but it seems short-sighted to ignore that, as Vida's caregivers, we also need to be OK.

Parents of unwell children go through a dramatic career change, becoming, among other things, activists and specialist nurses, on top of everything else that having a child brings. I have had to learn to accept a wildly different reality from the one I was expecting, adapting to unforeseeable routines and often maddening systems. Most of all, I have had to learn advocacy. For Vida, and for myself.

—

My hunch is that therapy can only do so much for me at this stage. 'We can't go over it! We can't go under it! Oh no! We've got to go through it,' go the lines in *We're Going on a Bear Hunt*, which come to me often over these months. I am swept up in the chaos of a hurricane, and I suspect I will only find perspective on its pressures and circulations when it slows.

For this reason, I only go to see Mandy – without Vida – a handful of times. She is a psychotherapist who has come recommended by a friend of my mum's and I like her instantly. Often I can't find the words for things, but she affirms my efforts to speak analytically. The good schoolgirl in me is encouraged by this and I feel myself wanting to do well for her. One of Mandy's mantras is that 'we suffer alone and we heal in relationship'. Her work, she says, is all about 'undoing aloneness'. I tell her I am surrounded by love and support but that I have never felt so alone. I would like my aloneness to be undone.

She suggests that Freddie comes to one of the sessions. He does, and it is there, with the levelling presence of an impartial third party, that I see where he is. He tells Mandy about his dad. He tells her about the months he spent in hospital, about the hope that he would recover and the real progress he made. He tells her about the sudden end.

'I thought I'd paid my dues,' he says.

Freddie is clear: Vida's diagnosis is a different thing – it *is* different, it *feels* different. It's that old thing about the natural order, about how a sick child tests the universal assumption that parents die first. Or maybe it is the responsibility – he is the father this time, making the decisions with me that will shape our daughter's life. Or maybe it's to do with the different ways we love the people that we love, about his fierce instinct to protect his baby and his limited ability to do so. I can't change any of this for Freddie. But I can do better than I have been. I have weight to pull in bringing our trajectories together. In the decisions we make for our child, we are two minds who must learn to act as one.

It will be three years before I'm in a position to speak to Mandy again, when I will have new perspective. This handful of early sessions were helpful, though, starting a process of undoing the aloneness that Freddie and I had each been feeling, even while going through the motions of having a baby, and then a diagnosis, together.

Vida is screeching in her high chair, naked except for a nappy, and banging her fists on the kitchen table: a Flintstone baby in Pampers, eating neon-orange puree. It's mango pulp that's caused this ruckus; Vida's gone wild for it. She cries out urgently, we scoop and sweep the spoon towards her open mouth and are met with the sound of 'Mmmmm'.

She's never been so excited about food before. Though her parents are gannets, the type of people that sit down for supper and talk about what they'll eat tomorrow, she's been largely unbothered by food so far. I have difficulty relating.

But this sudden delight, this joy, at a flavour – *this* I can relate to, and I am gagging to make it happen again. Mashed banana and porridge; the pleasure of a really mature Cheddar; her first suck on a string of spaghetti, *Lady and the Tramp* style;

fat rounds of cucumber, plain oatcakes, and sweet potato fries dunked in ketchup (watch her or she'll pick up the plate and lick it); Marmite pasta, Marmite rice cakes, Marmite on toast; berries and peaches in summer, apples and pears in autumn, clementines in winter; her inaugural portion of fish and chips, a blitzed-up Sunday roast: I revel in making these introductions, in being privy to those first jolts of pleasure or revulsion, the orchestrator of another human's relationship with taste.

When Vida eats, I sit with her, sometimes eat with her, always look at her. Mealtimes are, I discover, the perfect opportunity to practise the eye contact that the Hampstead therapist keeps mentioning, to sing to her, to chat to her, to watch her responses – and her to watch mine, my expressions encouraging her experiments in food. To feed her something she likes is the greatest triumph; to see her mastering a new skill – drinking from a cup, or through a straw, or lifting a spoon to her lips – beats any career landmark; to hear a *num-num-num* or a *mm-hmm-mm* feels like a round of applause that will never lose its thrill.

Away from hospitals, from Google, from other babies, food becomes a routine that dilutes the cordial of my terror. There's no lady I'd rather lunch with than this one.

Autumn arrives. After a summer spent swimming against a current of flaunted skin and high spirits, I am relieved by the change of season. Perhaps we never get over the sense of renewal that comes with a new school year. In any case, I feel more in tune with the cooler air, the shedding trees and the retreat of people into their homes.

Vida remains resistant to napping in her cot, so I pass many hours pacing around north London with the buggy, nearly always staying out for hours after she has woken up. Moving my body keeps my thoughts moving, too.

The days draw in and Halloween approaches. Our neighbourhood has particularly elaborate displays of spookiness, way above and beyond the carved pumpkins of my childhood. There are *Stranger Things* outfits, skeletons hanging from bay windows, even dogs in costume. Beyond West Hampstead, we march south, past the villas of Swiss Cottage and into Primrose Hill, where we wave to the giraffes peeking out of London Zoo and, one time, an escaped macaw. We walk along the canal in Little Venice, where some of the barges have started to light their wood burners, sending curls of smoke above us. Past the mannered calm of Maida Vale's Iyengar Yoga Institute, the illuminated flats of Elgin Avenue, where couples hunker down beneath their cornices, and up to Kilburn High Road, with its shishas and plastic bowls of fruit. So many side-by-sides, diversity and disparity, dynamic and troubling: Queen's Park's gourd displays and heavy front doors, a *Justice4Grenfell* tag never far away.

Off and on, I've lived in north-west London for longer than anywhere else in my adult life, but always at my mother-in-law Louise's house. My parents have a photo of my brother and me aged about seven and five, taken late one night in the 1990s, when instead of going to bed we had ransacked their wardrobes. Standing under an umbrella, I wear *The Lion King* pyjamas with my dad's enormous leather jacket hanging over the top, and my feet swim in a pair of Mum's heels. Living in West Hampstead feels a bit like that, like dressing up at home, assuming a grown-up life that I'm not quite ready for. Much of my psychic geography for this wedge of London is probably a bit fetishistic, composed of things I have read or watched and loved – Zadie Smith, Martin Amis, Viv Albertine, Zoë Heller, Richard Curtis.

Living here is helping me on several levels. Practically, it is close to Freddie's work, and we have Louise's support.

Physically, in removing me from Lewisham, which is dogged with difficult memories. Imaginatively, letting me pretend, a little, that I am someone else.

Today Vida and I are walking up to Hampstead. Mum was thrilled when I told her we were going to church, but I hasten to add that we aren't going, you know, *like that*.

I've heard through the grapevine about a singing group for babies and children in a church on Heath Street. It's free and, she assures me, not religious. She has cottoned on to the fact that I like singing to Vida and that Vida responds well when I do. The therapist Vida and I have been seeing together is emphatic about me needing to surround my daughter with language and to deliver it with eye contact. Singing has come to me more naturally than talking to her – perhaps its performative aspect takes me outside of myself, while talking to her all the time, as I've seen other mums do, requires natural extroversion beyond my current powers. But under duress, I eventually go.

The entrance is packed with buggies. People trickle in – mums and babies, nannies and their charges, the odd NW3 dad doing his bit – and walk past the font onto a small platform and towards a door from which, when it opens, the sound of a harmonica spills out. I pick Vida up and she peers around like a meerkat, looking for the source of the sound.

The small back room is full of people, many of them babies and toddlers jumping around in anticipation. There is a trio of musicians who wouldn't look out of place in Nashville but don't look quite so at home in Hampstead: the pastor, with a handlebar moustache, strums a guitar, singing an introductory number while people come in; a younger, very tall man is on the double bass; and an old dude – Gandalf meets Hell's Angel – plays a banjo. Their repertoire spans 'Daydream Believer' to 'Oats and Beans and Barley Grow', and the Sleeping Bunnies' theme tune to 'Old MacDonald'.

I feel my apprehensions melt away. Essentially, we've come to a performance. No introducing ourselves, no phones or snacks or chats while the music happens. Interaction is only with the trio and their instruments: stylophone, accordion, lap-steel guitar, toy piano, Ghanaian drum. We are spectators, safe, singing along when we feel like it. Which we – or I – do. It feels good. Vida, too, is rapt. I wish Freddie were here to witness the musicianship and, well, the joy. It feels extraordinary to enjoy something so ordinary as a music group with my baby.

Then sadness tugs at me – DBA never lets me have good moments for long. As C. S. Lewis wrote of his grief, 'Then comes a sudden jab of red-hot memory and all this "common-sense" vanishes like an ant in the mouth of a furnace.' I look around the room, imagining that beneath their natty clothes, skin, flesh, tissue, and within their bones, these children all have functioning bone marrow. But then I glance down at Vida, sitting perkily on my lap. She is doing everything all the other eight-month-old babies do. I am acutely aware of our difference, but also of our sameness.

In her excellent book *The Cracks that Let the Light In*, Jessica Moxham coins the phrase 'slanted motherhood' in reference to parenting her disabled son. To have a child with additional needs is motherhood experienced at a different angle, she says; particularly so, I think, when it is your firstborn and you have no 'normal' experience to compare it to. It is a curious vantage point – sometimes sad, but often powerful. It might be too soon to say that I feel empowered by Vida's diagnosis, but I am slowly acquiring a fresh perspective.

In between two songs, I get talking in whispers to the woman next to me, also with a baby on her knee. I still find mum chat difficult without caveating what has happened for us, and I tell her briefly about the blood disorder, the transfusions, all the things that haven't been as I expected. She listens intently and kindly. 'You wouldn't know,' she says.

The conversation is short – 'Do-Re-Mi' has begun – and I never learn her name. The exchange is significant, though. I already know that Vida doesn't 'wear' her invisible condition, but, clearly, I do. I realise that DBA really can be a detail in our lives; we can't control its existence, but we can control how much it pervades daily life.

Eight months into parenthood, Old Time Nursery (as the music group is called) gives Vida and me a public face as a mother-daughter pair. It satisfies my need for movement, for noise, for people, without the pressure of catching up with a friend to churn up recent history. Twice a week we go and get lost in music.

Freddie and I know better what to expect of transfusion days now, but so, I think, does Vida.

Cannulation involves at least four adults to hold her limbs and find a vein, keeping her as still as possible so they can draw blood before attaching the line, then to apply the dressing, the bandage, the splint. Often, Freddie will insist on going with Vida and the nurses to do the cannula in a treatment room away from our bay, sparing me. He has something to prove to himself, too, I think, after how terrible he'd found cannulation at Lewisham. A paediatric registrar had told him that he was making the situation worse for Vida when he became distressed. He had been troubled by the remark, and now makes sure he accompanies her to be cannulated every time we go to the Evelina. It seems heroic to me, this stepping into the furnace of his trauma and meeting it head-on. I sit on the bed, knees up, ready to pull out a boob to comfort Vida when she emerges with a bandaged arm.

These days can be very long. The haematology nurse has said that it might be better for us to come in for a blood test on one day – to do a 'cross match' between Vida and the donor's blood – and then to return the following day for the transfusion. This would supposedly save us waiting around, but I am put off by 1) an extra visit to hospital, and 2) an extra needle procedure.

We opt to do it all in a day, arriving at Snow Fox by 9 a.m. We insert the cannula, they take the blood, then Freddie and I take Vida to the South Bank until the blood-test results are back. We drink coffee and waft around cultural centres, anxiously second-guessing her haemoglobin level, until we get the call from one of the nurses to tell us that the blood has arrived on the ward. Her HB value determines how much blood she needs and how long the transfusion will be. Usually it is between two and three hours while she is this little, but the whole day can total twelve hours out of the house.

More and more, I can manage the day if getting through the transfusion is all that's required of me. The fact of Vida's DBA and the necessity of its treatment allow me to take an almost perfunctory approach to being in hospital. There is no choice involved; it's what we must do to keep her safe; we are getting to know the faces and the routine; we get home and that's it for another three weeks. *Bish bash bosh.*

But, while we are in hospital for Vida's transfusions, the normal lives of others go on, with their Doodle polls and dinner plans. I have masterfully avoided social encounters in recent months, but sometimes news of other people is inescapable. WhatsApp groups allow me to watch quietly what others are doing from a hospital bed while Vida sleeps. Baby sensory classes, flat whites, new haircuts. I deleted Instagram during Vida's emergency hospital admission, when an acquaintance with a newborn baby posted a picture of herself breezily breastfeeding at a fancy restaurant and looking immaculate, and I experienced a sort of implosion. It has been a relief to be spared those glimpses of the perfect lives of virtual strangers, but WhatsApp has stepped in with an equivalent offering, this time with the lives of those closer to us. I don't delete it because it's how I will stay in touch with them. It's also how I am staying in touch with the other DBA parents I have met – so it is something of a lifeline.

There's a particularly bittersweet transfusion day when an old friend's baby is born. I remember that high. Louise picks us up from the hospital and I sit next to Vida in her car seat, as she falls asleep holding my little finger. As we drive down the Mall, up Park Lane and onwards home down the Edgware

Road, I cry silently in the back while the others plan a meal I know I will not eat.

Freddie and I have always loved going away. We do it well. We are travellers led by our stomachs; meals on holiday are never incidental and usually thoroughly researched. Before, I had relished making our itineraries, but over the summer, when I had been unable to take to anything with either efficiency or interest, Fred stepped in as the family travel agent. He is clear in his determination to keep doing the things that make life enjoyable, mostly eating and drinking. It's time to go away and do both, he says.

We go to Berlin and stay in a trendy hotel, which is a ridiculous thing to do with a seven-month-old baby and gives us a first taste of holidays with kids. The scenic rooftop is off-limits after noon. There are loud media parties that come booming up the concrete pillars at night. After Vida's bedtime, Freddie and I tiptoe around with negronis to prove that we still can, then regret it when one of the parties wakes Vida up in the small hours. Our temples boom in unison with the pillars.

By day, though, the change of scenery is a relief. We wheel Vida around the city for hours on end. We eat sweet cinnamon buns for breakfast and drink strong coffee as we go. It's a weekend of full sensations, from the stark autumn light that casts geometric shadows across buildings to the stuttering movement of the buggy on cobbles, and the soaring in my heart when I see Vida in her swimming costume for the first time. She giggles when she catches me smiling at her. After months of mental stasis, movement comes in many forms, and it feels good.

We've been living at Louise's house for four months now and decide during these days in Berlin that we will sell our flat in Lewisham. It was an inevitability that had been growing with Vida, hardly the ideal space for the toddler she will soon become. But I have also become resistant to the idea of going back there. Just as some music has become unbearable – that Prince song, for instance, 'The Most Beautiful Girl in the World', from Vida's earliest days, or 'The Farmer's in His Den', which we had played endlessly out of a Fisher Price toy radio to try and calm her cries of distress – so too has the thought of those rooms where our baby was slowly losing her hold on life.

To my mind, our flat is, then, somewhere like a crime scene. I am viscerally opposed to moving back, and that feeling is reinforced on the few occasions we visit to pick up post and water the plants. Uninhabited, it smells cold; with the bottle steriliser on the kitchen counter and the bedside cot unmade in our room, it is a relic of another era. The lemon tree outside is flourishing, however. Its fruit is turning yellow and it is the picture of health. I am amazed that so neglected a plant is thriving. I find it faintly hopeful; I know better than to look for signs these days, but there is something reassuring about nature's onward march.

We find a new place to live, a few streets away from the flat. Close enough to feel familiar, but without some of the painful associations. It's a tiny, terraced house on a street sandwiched between two parks. Being that bit further from the high street and the station means there's more of a sense of community: there is a street WhatsApp group, we get to know our neighbours before we move in, there are more families.

The house needs a lot of love, but rather than dread the upheaval of building work, we eagerly take to planning for it. Both of us find it a welcome distraction; in the evenings, we lie in bed plotting. Freddie sketches floor plans on the backs of Vida's clinic letters while I trawl eBay for salvaged basins. I particularly enjoy dreaming up Vida's bedroom, the nursery we'd never got round to finishing at the flat. I choose bookshelves for her, a colour scheme to complement the curtain fabric we bought while I was pregnant (still in its box under the spare bed), a mobile of paper birds. This will be a new space to make our own, a secure base for our next chapter and whatever it brings.

At the end of September, we go to Cornwall with our parents. We stay in a house set on some cliffs in Gorran Haven, an ancient fishing village on the south coast. We walk, we cook, we spend a lot of time looking out to sea. I am also able to read, something I had come to believe I might never do for pleasure again. Not that it's pleasurable, exactly – my choice of material remains myopic – but I actively go searching for hopeful stories. A relatively new friend with both personal experience of ill health and an interest in psychology recommends that I read about 'post-traumatic growth', which I'm open to believing might be possible.

I also read a piece by a writer called Aleksandar Hemon in the *New Yorker*, titled 'The Aquarium', which is Hemon's account of his daughter's death. It chimes with my own impatience with spiritual platitudes; 'One of the most despicable religious fallacies is that suffering is ennobling,' he says, and I agree. But my daughter is alive and in the next room, gurgling in appreciation of blitzed-up roast chicken served with a sea view. *She* isn't suffering; she has moved on from that, and loves life, in spite – and possibly even because – of the extreme low she reached back in May. She is an emblem of post-traumatic growth, and all the enlightenment I will need to get better.

Freddie plunges into a grey wave with a half dive, turns quickly onto his back, pushing water forward with his palms, and gestures to me to join him. True to form, I'm barely knee deep. I always choose the painful approach, inching my way underwater at an agonising pace.

It's a cold September and the water is unappealing, but I'll regret it if I don't get in; there's something sacrilegious about being beside the sea and not having a dip. I am suddenly furious that Freddie has made the transition from land to water so easily, and in a flash I do it, submerging hips, shoulders, head.

You couldn't call it a swim, but as I run back to our towels, the wind hitting pearls of brine on my skin, I feel the sting of wellbeing.

Having another child has become my mission. We'd always assumed we'd have more than one, although perhaps not this quickly. I've heard other people speak of grabbing hold of life, surrounding themselves with it, in the wake of trauma. Rather than continuing to hide from life, I now feel myself looking for it, full of purpose. It feels like something tangible I can do to help Vida, too; not to mention myself, as, once again, it is something which gives me the illusion of control.

We meet with an embryologist at our chosen fertility clinic. This clinic is famous for its stellar success rates and is perhaps more familiar than most with what we need to do: PGD for HLA (human leukocyte antigen) typing. This is IVF with an extra layer of intervention: once embryos have been made, they can be tested using highly specialised probes that look for their sibling's genetic markers to make sure their stem cells 'match'. Like the conditions that it can help to treat, this kind of fertility treatment is rare. It is wondrous and technical stuff – and hugely expensive. It is not offered on the NHS.

The fact that any of this science is possible astounds me, but as impressed by it as I am, it still holds disappointment, for there are no guarantees. Because we are being extra-selective about the embryos, our odds of successfully getting a matched sibling are considerably slimmer than in ordinary IVF. How many eggs will they be able to get from me? Will any embryos survive their first few days, not to mention the subsequent testing, freezing and transfer processes? Will implantation work? Will any of them even be a match? We would probably find an unrelated match for Vida on the bone-marrow register, but the literature suggests that a matched sibling donor would make for the highest chances of a successful transplant. Also, she would only be allowed a transplant from an unrelated donor after all other options had been exhausted. If Vida has a BMT, I think, I'd rather it wasn't a desperate measure.

I trawl through articles online, many of them dating back to the mid-noughties, when the HFEA started granting licenses to do this kind of IVF to families like ours. The language is stirring, with terms like 'designer babies' and 'saviour siblings'. I find both to be problematic.

Before Vida's diagnosis, I had little experience of medicine, let alone medical ethics. Now I am knee-deep in finding solutions for my daughter, and it hadn't occurred to me that anyone might object to treatment like this. The ethics are surely that it's bloody fantastic. This could give my daughter a better life. An independent one, unencumbered by regular hospital visits and the many complications transfusion dependency brings.

Our second child will not be a 'designer baby'. We aren't talking about choosing an embryo based on eye or hair colour, or sex, indulging an aesthetic preference or a sexist predilection. Our child will be a much-wanted family member who happens to have a trait that could help their sister in a way no one else could. We want to give Vida the best chance we can. Who could possibly argue with that? (Plenty of people, it turns out, but I limit my exposure to them, keeping my echo chamber small and validating.)

If 'designer baby' swipes at the parents, 'saviour sibling' loads responsibility onto the child that results from this kind of IVF. No child of ours will be a saviour sibling – we know that, but we don't want these words to be used by anyone else, either. A matched sibling *could* change the course of things for Vida, but it won't be their duty to do so – if they don't, or if it doesn't work, there is no failure on their part.

Even with a perfectly matched sibling donor, bone-marrow transplants are complex medical procedures, not divine interventions, as the word 'saviour' would imply. We are on the side of the mortals – this has never been clearer to me. It is no one else's responsibility to save us, but medicine can help. And we're calling on it.

I've heard it said that the mind is the strongest muscle. And I believe this to be true. But, like legs, bums and tums, the mind contains many muscles, some of them stronger than others. It needs exercise and repeated use to become powerful.

As soon as we knew something was not right in Vida's bone marrow, I committed my brain to theory, reading and rereading papers that could enlighten us about what might be happening. It has been quite the mental workout. Until now, I've rarely had to make important decisions in my life. This situation demands pragmatism, and pragmatism requires patience – something I definitely do not have. I want a solution. I want to make Vida better. Fast.

I must accept that nothing will happen quickly. This is not an attitude that comes naturally to me, so it's unsurprising that I find the slowness of progress a form of torture. Freddie is a proponent of 'one step at a time', breaking down the almighty task into smaller ones. I just wish I found this easier.

I am more comfortable with hatching grand plans about bone-marrow transplants and having another baby than engaging in talk about some of the medications that Vida is likely to need imminently. Some of this is because I like the idea of liberating her from regular hospital visits (the ordeal of transplant notwithstanding – about this I am still very naive). But more than this, there's a part of me that is trying to think my way out of this for Vida, for us. It's a coping mechanism of sorts. Being in my head about the whole thing – planning, scheming – is, I suspect, keeping sadness at bay, a sadness that can otherwise threaten to engulf me.

I am also aware, however, that I mustn't project that sadness onto Vida. Not only must I stop seeing myself as a victim here, but I need to resist the idea that Vida is one. When she looks into my eyes, I want her to see peace reflected. The knowledge that she is entirely who and what she is supposed to be. I remind myself every day that I wouldn't have Vida if she didn't have DBA, and with that in mind, pragmatism starts to feel more possible.

So it is around this time that I choose pragmatism. As Freddie has kept saying, I have the power to decide how I respond to this. I can value this thing that has caused me pain because it has given me my daughter – *this* feisty daughter, who cackles with delight every night when Freddie flings her over his shoulder and I chase them up the stairs to the bathroom. It is a joy so pure that I am rendered utterly unoriginal in my assessment of it. It lights up my world.

—

I am starting to think about writing, sensing the need for an outlet beyond therapy. I'm not someone who trusts my own instinct before I've thrashed it out on a keyboard. But, of course, opportunities for this have been scarce since Vida was born.

During our buggy walks, I've thought a bit about how to frame the experience I've had of new motherhood, conscious of how writers like Amy Liptrot and Raynor Winn gave shape to their troubles through the lens of, respectively, nature and walking. But I quickly abandon the idea, knowing that it is too soon. I am as yet too much within the maelstrom to give it a clear voice or meaningful resolution – or any meaning whatsoever. I still wrestle with the absolute meaninglessness of a sick child.

Plus, words – always my currency of choice – seem a poor representation for everything I feel. I'm not alone in feeling this way; after I told her what had happened, one friend, a writer and a mother, wrote to me, 'Words fail.' Briefly I'd felt annoyed that she hadn't found them, but I couldn't either, so, fair enough, I concluded.

Will I ever be able to write this time faithfully? If I can find words that approximate it, the order inherent to a sentence will surely belie the chaos of it all.

Still, I sense the stirrings of creativity and act on them. I go to the art shop in Hampstead and buy a sketchbook, a 4B pencil and a rubber. I haven't drawn more than the odd doodle in a notepad since school but, when I start sketching before bed at night, I'm reminded of how transportive it can be. I start with Freddie, tracing his profile illuminated by his laptop screen. Like writing, it is a process that gives rise to what I didn't know I knew: my husband's deep-set eyes, his strong, almost geometric nose, his tense, thinking mouth. Unlike when I write, I don't really think. Drawing puts me in a state of not-thinking.

I move on to drawing Vida. This is impossible to do from life, so I use photos, which always result in her looking like a ventriloquist's doll. Her milky features, so soft, offer no hooks or angles to the pencil in my hand. The upshot is rather haunting, but the process of studying her features in this way feels important; I think about the person behind them. And in her soulful, dark-rimmed green eyes, above those peachy cheeks and pursed lips, I see her spark.

Towards the end of October, one of my therapist Mandy's mottos – 'We suffer alone, we heal in relationship' – is put to the test. Or, rather, it is affirmed. Not only are Freddie and I more of a team, but I am reminded of the life-giving quality of friends.

My friend Nick, who I met during my year abroad in America, is getting married this month. Studying abroad as not-quite adults makes for cast-iron friendships, and mine with Nick and the third in our trio, Holly, is one such. We formed something like a family during that time and now, nearly fifteen years after we met, Holly and I are, respectively, Nick's reader and witness at his and his partner Rob's small ceremony in south London.

Our friend Lily comes over from Los Angeles for the wedding. She is staying with us and arrives a few days early to spend some time together. I am apprehensive about having a house guest, given my early bedtimes and antisocial tendencies; will she recognise me?

But Lily is one of the people with whom I can run the gamut of conversation, from hot sauce to paediatric wards, because she has experienced something comparable – albeit as a patient herself. Lily was diagnosed with Hodgkin lymphoma in her late teens and was treated with some of the drugs that Vida will likely need one day, too. She took time out of school for intensive treatment and returned a term later in remission. This was when I met her. She was on the board of a philanthropic theatre group, a charismatic, pixie-haired young woman with a killer dress sense, never not surrounded by people and always laughing. It was only later that I learnt what she'd been through.

I tell her about how I have been looking for other people's stories, how there are so few of them, how what I need isn't even so grand as hope, but to feel less alone in my new role as the mother of a patient. She tells me about a short story she once read by Lorrie Moore, 'People Like That are the Only People Here', written from the perspective of a mother on a paediatric oncology ward after her child's sudden and devastating diagnosis. It's in a short-story collection called *Birds of America*, which I order immediately; it arrives the next day.

Reading this story is like coming home – what a relief to read my own thoughts, thoughts which have been had by someone else before, in all their mania and dark humour. From the narrator's addiction to 'the sadness and emergencies of others' to, in her disbelief at the diagnosis, wondering where 'chemotherapy' and 'Hickman catheter' were in the indexes of all the baby books she'd read. Never had fiction so resembled my life. There is fear and wisdom in its pages, and it crystallises my thoughts. Because, yes, exactly this: 'Look at all the things you have to do to protect a child, a hospital merely an intensification of life's cruel obstacle course.'

Life intensified. But life it still is. I guzzle the story. I never could have imagined feeling upbeat after reading something like this. But that, I suppose, is the power of kinship – even with a fictional character. Lorrie Moore's story also feels like therapy. She points out how the horror of childhood illness has proportions almost too epic for the page.

It reminds me of something I once heard on the radio about why Donald Trump is so difficult to satirise; you can't push such a character to further extremes. Similarly, the brutality of serious childhood illness sits at the end of the line – unsubtle, unimaginable. Who wants to write that? Let alone read it.

Perversely, though, I feel emboldened to put pen to paper. Once Lily leaves a week later, I start.

On Nick and Rob's wedding day, Vida stays at home with Louise. I go to Camberwell to help get the venue ready with Holly and Lily. Leaving the house without my daughter is thoroughly disorienting. I feel like a dropped yo-yo; my momentum gone, I become a different, simpler, thing.

And I enjoy it! We drink sparkling wine and write place settings, put on makeup and take photographs together before the booze deglazes our faces. In the town hall, I hold hands with Freddie and Holly as we watch our friends say their vows. Nick's voice has a texture I've never heard before. Love soars over the room. *We heal in relationship.*

The wedding marks a significant step forward. I feel like something close to myself among people I love and doing some of the things I used to like – and still do, I discover – eating and drinking, dancing and talking. There is lightness to the day after many months of feeling like a dead weight.

It was also the first day of measurable change in my IVF efforts. As we sit down for lunch, I look at my phone and see that there's an email from our specialist nurse: she has sent me the letter from Josu confirming Vida's diagnosis and the possibility of bone-marrow transplant further down the line. I'd been anxiously waiting for this, a vital tool in our application to the HFEA. And here it is – in a moment when I happen to be raising a glass, no less. My eyes meet Freddie's across the table. I feel such relief: now we can make progress. For the first time in far too long, I really tuck into a meal.

The IVF clinic will now be able to apply for a licence to perform HLA typing on our behalf, giving the clinic special permission to select an embryo based on its genetic suitability. In other words, if we are lucky, we will have a baby who we know to be a match for Vida. We are one step closer to having our second child.

A happy day becomes happier. But this, I think now, is remarkable, given the content of the letter: 1,297 words outlining the gravity of the process she will go through if she has a bone-marrow transplant: six days of chemotherapy, with all its well-known side effects; a 'period of neutropenia' of around six weeks, during which we would live in an air-filtrated isolation cubicle; and a period of immunosuppression of at least six months, when patient, parents and medical team alike sit in anxious suspense at the possibility of graft-versus-host disease (GvHD), a condition where the donor cells attack the recipient's. Josu once again reels off statistics of probabilities, possibilities, likelihoods.

Medical letters don't spare your feelings. It's almost surprising that they are intended for the patient's or parents' eyes. At times their clipped sentences feel like an attack, with their ugly symbols and conservative take on hope. If you really can't be more positive, I think, then why bother treating her at all?

But then, of course, I am also infuriated by other people's positivity. Truthfully, I appreciate being levelled with. This letter may be hard to read, but it tells it like it is: DBA is tough, but there are the things we can try. There is hope. I'm not sure we can ask for much more than that.

While I have hungrily sought out other people's experiences, I haven't really offered any of my own. I've avoided engaging with the Diamond-Blackfan community because participation would feel too much like acceptance. Those I *have* spoken to are DBA elders, with hopeful stories and motivational wisdom that nursed me through the summer. And then, of course, Al Gilmour and his wife Emily, who I contacted because the proximity of our worlds seemed so bizarre – there was comfort and strength in numbers, albeit a very small number. Masha Gessen puts this well in her book *Blood Matters*: 'Each new flesh-and-blood acquaintance made my predicament seem less extreme,' she says, of finding a community of other women in her shoes. (Gessen has a mutation on the BRCA1 gene, which brings with it an inflated predisposition to breast and/or ovarian cancer. Actor Angelina Jolie has this too, and famously had an elective mastectomy to offset some of the risk of breast cancer developing.)

All this time, I have lurked on the fringes of the DBA UK charity Facebook page, a ghoulish spectator. The page is a closed group for patients, parents and, in some cases, other family members, where people share their progress, research, fundraising, worries and questions. It seems to offer solace to many parents, but so far I have not been one of them. I wouldn't know these people were it not for Vida having DBA, and I don't want her to be defined by it. Forming friendships out of it feels wrong, somehow forced, a declaration of membership to something I hope she can transcend.

'Ya'll are the best,' someone has written, after several other parents have chimed in with advice on a DBA-related problem. 'So grateful for this group,' many say. I find the gratitude alienating now, but I will soon see the value of social media. How else could I be connected to this many other families in a similar position? Over time, I will find comfort in the shorthand between the DBA families on Facebook, a place where acronyms don't need spelling out; where words like *reticulocyte* and *erythroblast* are the vernacular; where people really grasp the concerns we face, because they share them. Facebook will eventually normalise an existence with which no one I know 'in real life' is familiar. In the early days, I am terrified by the things I read on it; later, with my acceptance, its community will be a tonic.

Already I have read things written by other parents that have helped to explain some of Vida's quirks, like her declining appetite over the three weeks between transfusions. In the realm of the rare, where research is lean, sharing individual experience is vital. It helps to build a body of knowledge and to shape lives for the better. Realising this is a turning point and I decide to buckle up and make my first post. Many parents introduce themselves with a photo of their child and short summary of their DBA journey to date. I do just this with a picture of Vida now, aged seven months. She looks adorable in her pink puffa and a bobble hat, her face with a hint of her dad's 'signature frown', a look of deep thought.

I am starting to recognise names in the group, too. One is Zoe, who I had read about before Vida had even been diagnosed. Zoe had contacted the Sandcastle Trust – a charity which gives experiences to families with children suffering genetic conditions, of which I am now a trustee – when her son, who has DBA, was a toddler. They'd given him a year's membership to Colchester Zoo. He'd loved it, visiting regularly to see the penguins, which Zoe had written about for the charity's blog. At the time, I had skim-read it and promptly closed the page, horrified both by the thought of the gorgeous blonde boy I saw in the pictures being 'hooked up' to a needle and pump to remove excess iron every night and by the fact that his mum had to give up work to take care of him full time.

Then, in July, when I had been waiting to go into our first clinic appointment with Josu, I had seen that same little boy with his mother. He had recently had a transplant, his hair only starting to grow back, but he looked like a happy, bouncy kid in spite of what he was going through. I also remember the warmth that exuded from his mum. I didn't say hello – but

I probably did her a favour. At the time I had been prone to leeching off sages like her.

In the intervening months I have followed their post-transplant journey online. It isn't a smooth ride and, as they are strictly in isolation, social media is proving a bit of a lifeline for Zoe. One evening in early October, I write to her on a whim. I tell her I've been following her story and that Vida was diagnosed with DBA earlier this year. She writes back quickly, a furnace of gratitude for my getting in touch. I am so glad I have done this. Over the following weeks, we busily exchange messages (sometimes nearly novella-length) to build a picture of each other's position – how our children came to be diagnosed, how they are doing now and, vitally, how we each have coped.

A clinical psychologist, Zoe is both versed in unpicking medical-speak and a champion of empathy. She has researched DBA even more zealously than I have and is hot on research developments. She is generous with her learnings, advising me on how to navigate milestones from steroids to chelation, bone-marrow biopsy to MRI. And most of all, she is also a mother who has faced the possibility of losing her child to a condition so nuanced that it's sometimes impossible to believe in, especially when it's mostly invisible. We won't meet in person or see each other's faces except in photos for another two years, but I feel more seen by her than almost anyone else. And I feel hopeful that, in time, I might be able to gather myself as she has.

Around the same time, I get a message from a woman in America, Lauren. Her profile picture is a family selfie taken in a golf buggy, all four of them – a mother, a father and two girls, one of them a baby – with bronzed skin and beautiful smiles.

Her fifteen-month-old daughter, the baby in the photo, was recently diagnosed with DBA. She has seen the post I made about Vida. Her tone feels familiar; to someone not in our boat, her considered assembly of words might seem composed. To me, they betray a mother casting around for meaning in the face of the unknown. Like us, Lauren and her husband hadn't registered their daughter's paleness because its onset was slow, an ebbing away of colour that went undetected until a routine blood test picked up anaemia. She is still in deep shock.

Lauren's daughter is a few months older than Vida but more recently diagnosed, and in our early conversations, she grills me on what I know. It is the first time that someone further behind me in the process has been in touch. In these first days of chatting, I feel a flicker of competence; I am pleased to be able to put my experience to work in the form of pep talks which seem, briefly, to buoy us both. Shrilly, we look to the positives. The girls will be OK because they have us! We agree that things could be so much worse! But it doesn't take long before I confess how badly I've taken things, how DBA so baffles me that I can hardly believe it's a real illness. Manic positivity segues into shared despair, then back to a place of hope, we ride a pendulum that swings between the two. But we ride it together.

We message each other all the time, urgently, fiercely; together in our aloneness, in our severance from the security we thought we had. It feels like the kind of tight, exclusive girl friendships I had as a teenager. Mandy's 'undoing aloneness' feels real to me in these weeks, my own aloneness undone by knowing someone coping with a similar thing at a similar time. We are both struggling with the fearsome things we read on Facebook – matter-of-fact talk of failed steroids, congenital abnormalities, and the side effects of treatments – and I realise that it's not enough simply to know other parents dealing with the condition. Having another parent navigating the same stage is innately valuable, too.

Diamond-Blackfan is levelling. It has put me in contact with people I'd never have otherwise met, rendering the common ground I tend to share with friends – background, geography, politics, work – irrelevant. Now we have a new category: biology. For that is all this is, the random reorganisation of a tiny gene in a small, disparate number of babies around the world.

With both Lauren and Zoe, we talk only about DBA at first, but over time, develop friendships in their own right. I haven't chosen to know them, but genes dictate that I do, and with that comes a muddle of feelings – but also, an understanding. It's like family, really.

During this period of friend-making, I start to soften. I see how powerless some of our friends and family must have felt – powerless to remove my pain, and powerless even to offer any solace. Short of a change in the diagnosis, nothing in those early months could make me feel better. Grief is lonely for the griever and alienating for the people who love them. I understand this now.

Freddie, our mums and I start to be more prescriptive with friends about what would be helpful to us. We suggest that people join us for a transfusion day, as this will offer us company during the long hours in hospital, and perhaps give them a clearer idea of what Vida's condition involves. On transfusion days, there can be no living in denial – after three weeks without, her treatment is urgent – so they are technically the days when we might most feel the sting. I have learnt, though, that hospital days often aren't the hardest, surrounded as you are by upbeat professionals who are there to help. Instead, grief creeps up when my guard is down. Still, I really appreciate the show of support – spending a day on a paediatric ward isn't anyone's first choice for their annual leave, but people do it because they care.

On the whole, these are good days surrounded by our best allies. My brother, Max, and his girlfriend, Becky, meet us for coffee at the Royal Festival Hall while we wait for Vida's blood, then join us on the ward with some brownies, scrunching the paper bag and jangling their keys in a makeshift baby sensory session. Our friends Raffi and Grace meet us at the Tate Modern, where an installation offers Vida inflated and multiple versions of herself in a mirrored room. Pet, who arrived as our family au pair in 1998 and has been a surrogate sister ever since, flies in from Prague and comes straight to the hospital, sending us out for a walk while she plays with Vida. Katharine and Sophie, Vida's godmothers, both spend a day with us on Snow Fox, regularly scooping her up for a cuddle and masterfully navigating the line as they do so. Having my best friends around gives Freddie the chance to pop out for a breather, and me a cup of tea to sip slowly. As Vida feels the effect of haemoglobin in her system, she perks up and becomes restless; these days attached to a transfusion are a workout for Freddie and me, and extra help is welcome.

It is hard and deeply moving to see an infant attached to a blood transfusion. All these people come in strength, fortifying us with their love.

It's a Thursday afternoon in mid-November and I'm in the bath. Sometimes, if she has a gap between patients, Louise will take Vida for half an hour so I can, as she puts it, poach myself. I have always loved really hot baths – anything other than almost scalding seems pointless; there is pleasure in the pain of easing myself in, my skin quivering as it meets the water's heat.

My impatience with the IVF situation is reaching a crescendo. Everything in the world of fertility treatment ticks to the rhythm of the intended mother's menstrual cycle, and even small administrative delays, such as the post being slow, or a postponed meeting, can push treatment back by a whole month. We are waiting for a licence to do HLA typing from the HFEA, and I know that our case was being discussed in a committee meeting this week. On a whim, I call them from my bath, expecting another bump in the road.

To my surprise, the senior inspector managing our case tells me that the application has been approved today – in the last hour, no less. A green light after many reds and roadworks and sirens.

My pushiness now becomes directed at the clinic. I pester them for action. When will the probe, tailor-made to check for Vida's mutation, be ready? What can I do to prepare? Is there anything I can do to make myself as, well, as fertile as possible? I start having acupuncture and eat a lot of eggs, having gleaned from Mumsnet that both can help.

The clinic also tells me that my ovarian reserve is 'on the lower end of normal', which is the kind of knowledge I could really do without. I hear 'lower' much more loudly than I hear 'normal', and can't stop thinking about all my little eggs, inside me since birth, dwindling in number with every month we delay treatment.

While I had obviously hoped I could conceive naturally, as I did with Vida, I had taken for granted that IVF would be there for me if I needed it. Fertility's safety net. I know a few people who have had children via IVF but, until now, have thought little about what they had to go through to hold a baby of their own in their arms. I'm learning fast that this treatment is as emotionally brutal as it is a physical imposition, and I haven't even started it yet.

The whole thing is predicated upon failure. There's roughly a 25 per cent chance of conceiving in any cycle, assuming you can harvest enough eggs to work with. I will be given a cocktail of hormones to boost my ovaries into maturing a number of egg follicles – ideally between ten and twenty, when a standard month might give just one or two – which, when harvested, will meet Freddie's sperm in the eponymous *vitro*. Our chances of success are further impacted by the 25 per cent odds of getting the HLA match we're after. They'll have to get eggs from me, fertilise them, let them grow for five or six days, then test them for the match and freeze them. Any appropriate embryos – i.e. chromosomally balanced, and ideally HLA-matched to Vida – will then need to survive thawing before being put back inside me to, we hope, grow into a healthy pregnancy. It's the Grand National of conception.

We picked this clinic because they have the highest success rates in the industry. Unfortunately, they also seem to have the highest prices – but how can you put a price on a child? A much-wanted baby and a stem-cell match for Vida. Some women on the fertility forums liken the regimen to a boot-camp for the ovaries. It is, I am told, going to be profoundly stressful. We have the best doctors in the business overseeing the physiological side of things, but I am nervous of the toll this could take on my already fragile mind. How do women do this without going completely mad?

Given that old-fashioned sex sufficed before, I can't believe I'm jumping through all these hoops to have another child. A licence! Egg harvesting! Genetic testing! I feel like the protagonist of a sci-fi novel.

Together, Freddie and I have always taken a childish delight in Christmas. I'd assumed that events of the last year would've changed that. But twinkly December feels good for the soul.

Of course, things are different to what I'd imagined a year ago, but Vida's first Advent is nonetheless a happy time. I love wrapping her up in her snowsuit and seeing her breath make little puffs of steam on the cold air. I love marching up to Hampstead for the music group and noticing how she gazes at the white lights on streetlamps, the Christmas displays and Hanukah candles in windows. Seeing the constructs of the festive season through her eyes feels like a kind of magic.

We are speeding towards Vida's first birthday and I can see how her sense of self is emerging. She sits up comfortably, hurling herself forward at the hips and into crawling position.

She usually flops down at this point, but every day her suspension improves: it won't be long until she's on the move. She is adept, in her own brand of babble, at expressing how she feels about things. She loves anything on wheels, low-hanging Christmas-tree baubles, and her very favourite thing is a travel bottle of Louise's purple shampoo, which she tips up and down, mesmerised as the liquid moves.

Every meal is a multi-course affair designed to get her to eat; unlike my friends' babies – such as my friend Boo's son, who demolishes everything from hummus to curry, as I'd imagined my baby would – Vida is suspicious of food. Whether this comes from a contrary nature or having been forcibly prodded and fed things for so much of her life to date, I don't know, but getting her to eat from a spoon can be tricky. She prefers finger food, with a preference for grated cheese, pasta shells, broad beans and blueberries, which I burst in half with my teeth before handing them to her.

I have been told to stop breastfeeding before the IVF starts after Christmas – it can adversely affect your fertility, they say. Given the process is already costing us a lot of money, I decide to give it my all and spend the month slowing down on the feeds. I think I would feel more upset about this if I weren't so full of purpose about the IVF, but I do nonetheless feel a sentimental tug at the thought of giving up. We worked hard to get here, to a place where feeding felt as natural as I knew it could be. My depression and Vida's anaemia kept tripping us up in those early months, just as we were finding our groove. But breastfeeding has become a comfort to us both, softening the hard edges of distress on hospital days and broken nights, a union. I am wary of hospital days without it, especially given Vida's new mobility and increasingly loud objections to being tethered by the line.

In her first year I have felt the gradual extrication of my baby from my body. We remained part of one another long after she was born, and now, weaning her off breastmilk feels like a dramatic breaking of the tie. But her independence from my body in fact brings with it even greater connection between us. She makes a huge amount of noise and is unafraid of making herself known to the world. She hoots when Freddie hides behind the side of the bath when she is in it, popping his head up and wiggling his tongue; she despises being left too long in the pram or highchair, squawking with displeasure; she rolls over and cries out when we try to change her nappy. She demands constant entertainment. She has verve; Boo calls her a firecracker.

Sometimes I wonder whether she has DBA at all, because she seems the very antithesis of unwell. Every transfusion day, when we wait for her haemoglobin result to come back, I hold out for the possibility that her HB has held and her reticulocytes have shot up, signalling that elusive spontaneous remission we've heard about. This never happens, but her HB levels do vary quite wildly. One time it's as high as 120 (which isn't even classified as anaemic), and at others it's in the 80s, which we are told will definitely affect how she feels. Apparently this variation is probably due to the immense rate of growth during a baby's first year – Vida's need for and use of haemoglobin will change week by week.

I am becoming more seasoned at spotting the signs of anaemia in her, too. They can be very subtle, not least because transfusions take her levels higher than that of many healthy children. She is peachy with fresh blood, but gradually this colour fades over the three weeks; the cartilage at the top of her ears loses its pink glow, the flush wanes in her rosebud lips, she looks tired around her eyes. I feel more and more incredulous that we, and the various medics we saw in those early weeks, didn't see how ill she was. I look at the photos now and see only that – the yellowish hue, the hollow eyes. Sallow is the word, an appearance of shocking definition. And it did define her then – her look, her life – but it doesn't now. She is thriving and her character bursts forth.

It will take time for the weight I feel in my stomach and chest to lift, but sometimes I catch myself laughing. I wonder if it is appropriate to laugh. As I start to approach an even keel, I often police my feelings in this way. But haven't the last months been punishment enough without me punishing myself? I am allowed to laugh, and frankly, I can't help it. I have such a funny daughter.

It's Vida's last transfusion before Christmas and things have been a bit held up. Snow Fox is full of regular patients getting their final treatment of the year, and I imagine the whole of St Thomas' is fielding winter bugs. As somebody who relies on the hospital year-round, I struggle with this seasonal demand. This is probably a symptom of being institutionalised: feeling ownership of the place that keeps my daughter alive.

I have seen more of the nurses here than many of my family and friends this year; I look forward to seeing them, even if I still anticipate transfusion days with dread. 'Getting big!' Patrick often says when he hasn't seen Vida for three weeks.

She's started smiling at him in recognition. As much as any of our friends, the team at the Evelina are the people who are watching Vida grow. I feel immense warmth towards them. They know my daughter, anticipate her reactions, notice that her veins are getting bigger and therefore easier to access. They also know us, have doubtless noticed my tears and hot cheeks on some of the harder days, but never made a fuss, always dignifying my sadness with space and the offer of tea.

Today we waited a while before the cannula was put in, then the blood took a few hours to arrive, then the line kept occluding once her transfusion had started. This is increasingly a problem. When Vida was smaller, she'd sleep for up to half the transfusion, breastfeed, or look around while sitting on one of our laps. Now she wriggles, mouths and yanks at whatever is within her reach. (With tinsel and decorations hanging from every wall and ceiling, the ward during December is a veritable sweetshop for a ten-month-old.) Sometimes, if she moves her arm, it causes a kink in the line and the transfusion stops. A nurse will nip in and restart it, often for the same thing to happen again, and again.

Together with the Snow Fox gang, we have devised a two-pronged strategy to help avoid this happening. First, we put a baby splint on not just one but both sides of her elbow to hold it straight. Secondly, Freddie has taken to taping the line to Vida's back, so there's no visible slack for her to pull. I then put a piece of clothing over her – cardigans with balloon sleeves are the name of the game here.

Today we are watching Christmas episodes of *Hey Duggee* and *The Baby Club*. I sing 'Jingle Bells' to Vida, bouncing her gently on my knee while she sucks on a segment of tangerine.

One of the nurses looking after us pops into our bay. 'Do you need some Exjade?' she asks.

'Oh no, she doesn't take that yet,' I say, casually. The literature suggests starting iron chelation, to remove the dangerous build-up of the metal in the organs of transfusion-dependent patients, after about ten to fifteen transfusions. But Josu's plan is for her to try steroids first.

'It's just that her ferritin is high – the consultants usually chelate at this level.'

Until now, I haven't paid any attention to Vida's ferritin level, the blood protein that transports iron around the body – I only know to ask what her haemoglobin count is. But today confirms that she has iron overload. It seems absurd that all this metal is chugging around my daughter's bloodstream. I muse about whether she might be magnetic, then catch her eye and she smiles. *Yes*, I think, *magnetic you are*.

Iron is the grave side effect of ongoing transfusion therapy. So far I have been in denial about it, knowing we'll have to deal with it later. Typically, I always believe that Vida could be an exception to the rule, defying her condition. Maybe iron overload won't be a problem for her? Over and over, my hopefulness misfires like this – I need to learn how to hope within the bounds of what is possible.

Chelation therapy is the process by which a drug binds to metals in a patient's bloodstream and removes it through their urine. I've hated the word 'chelation' since I first heard it, how it creaks and crunches, as clunky as iron itself. All transfusion-dependent patients – DBA or otherwise – need treatment, which comes in two possible forms: a tablet or a pump, which is administered by caregivers, who insert a needle into their child before bed. This is hooked up to a device in a backpack or bumbag, which releases the drug while they sleep.

Several times people have kindly suggested we give her an iron supplement for her anaemia or sneak some liver into her food. Unlike the anaemia I had after her birth, Vida's anaemia is not caused by iron deficiency, and iron supplementation is not the answer. Quite the opposite. When she has a transfusion, she receives not just the donor's haemoglobin but the iron that comes with it.

I call our specialist nurse at St Mary's. Her iron is really high, I tell her.

'It will go high,' she says, 'but we won't need to do anything about it until the spring. I will speak to the team and explain.'

This is one of the intricacies of treating a rare condition in action. Vida's care is split between the Evelina – the children's hospital at St Thomas' – and St Mary's, the specialist centre for paediatric red-cell disorders in the UK. Brilliant as the team are at the Evelina, we need the expertise of St Mary's. They have to be in regular contact about Vida.

With permission to stay in denial for a little longer, we hold off on chelation for now. We finish Vida's transfusion after Snow Fox closes, on one of the Evelina's twenty-four-hour wards. There are children who have been here for weeks, who may even be in for Christmas. How lucky we are, I think, mostly to be outpatients. I don't think I would have been able to say or see that a few months ago.

—

'Plate!'

Freddie holds a small metal spatula and scraper which between them contain a glob of oozing cheese that he's melted under a tiny but fierce grill on the table. Our friend Beatrice holds out a plate with boiled baby potatoes and cornichons arranged on it, and Freddie flaps the cheese on top. We're serving our friend who lives in Switzerland (a very basic version of) something she can get anytime, anywhere in Geneva, but Fred was determined to use his new gadget. The raclette machine came out.

Throughout this year, Freddie has stayed determined to keep doing the things that he loves. 'It's how you deal with these things,' he so often says to me gently.

While I have scrolled through my phone, Freddie has spent much of the last few months constructively: he's gone to work, cooked, swooped Vida off for early-morning walks and researched all the stuff I don't seem to get to – bottle brands, nappy bins, age-appropriate bath toys – even baby sunglasses. He really makes her laugh in a way I can't. 'She thinks she *is* you, or that you're her,' says Louise. 'The booby prize . . . literally,' I say.

I have had moments of envying Freddie his ability to suspend some of the heavy feelings he's had this year. But watching him now, making raclette, sipping his drink, talking animatedly with our friend about grilling and pickles, I feel proud. He's drawing a line under a hard year in the best way he knows: potatoes, melted cheese, good people.

—

At the end of January, I start IVF. Louise has a tiny fridge in her cellar, used once a year for the influx of Christmas booze, but which we have kept switched on to house a panoply of fertility-boosting drugs.

I find I welcome the clinic's gruelling regimen – this level of face time with nurses is reassuring; the daily blood tests confirm that, after months of waiting, it's really happening. It feels rather chi-chi, nipping onto the Jubilee line and popping down to the Harley Street neighbourhood every day; I treat myself to books in Daunt and bougie cheese, and think I could get used to a Marylebone lifestyle... Admittedly, my purpose for being here is distinctly unglamorous. I used to feel squeamish when I had a blood test, but after months of watching needles go into my baby, I am hardened to the spectacle.

At the beginning of my IVF cycle, an internal scan reveals only a few visible follicles on my ovaries, which I am told should change after a few days of hormones. Three days in, the gynaecologist calls to tell me that my progesterone levels are not coming up fast enough; he prescribes a course of Clomid – a drug used to prompt ovulation. I do not need any more bumps in my childbearing road. Where are all my eggs?

Before going back to the *Guardian*, I have agreed to do some freelance work for the Waitrose food magazine as a contributing editor one day a week. It is a nice opportunity to dip my toe back into the world of work, and though joining a new team is in some ways daunting, it feels easier to establish myself anew here than to go back to my old job so fundamentally changed. This seems more like a warm-up, and a lovely one too, a team of mostly women, a different readership, a healthy budget, and a test kitchen that produces treats throughout the day. Food has become more appealing, not least from necessity; I've been told to eat lots of protein during IVF. I flex my food-editor muscles, putting together a feature about the history of chocolate for the Easter issue and brainstorming ideas to mark this year's seventy-fifth anniversary of VE Day.

After several false starts, we have recently found someone to look after Vida at Louise's house a few days a week. We start the arrangement a month before I go back to the *Guardian*, giving her and Vida time to settle with each other. In the early mornings I go to Marylebone for my blood test and, on the days I don't work, come home to lie on the bed alone. It would be restful, if only I couldn't hear the commotion downstairs. It hasn't been the smoothest transition because Vida can be tricky about both naps and meals. She also seems to miss me. When I enter the room after some hours apart, she cries out, affronted, in disbelief, riled and relieved, as if to say, 'Where the hell have you been?'

Truthfully, I don't find our separation straightforward either. I crave time to myself that, when I get it, is tainted by a longing for her. Time alone will never truly be time alone again – physically, maybe, but not psychically.

Another few days into IVF, and it is in the corridor at the Waitrose magazine office on Old Street where I receive a call from the gynaecologist. My body isn't responding to the drugs as they'd hoped. The way things are looking, they'll get no more than four eggs when they 'harvest' them in another few days.

They might not all fertilise, or make it to the five-day 'blastocyst' stage, or survive testing or freezing. It's also quite possible that none of them will be a match. And that's before all the usual uncertainty around IVF – will a pregnancy 'stick' if and when an embryo is transferred? He levels with me: probability suggests that we are unlikely to finish this process with the result we want – a stem-cell-matched sibling for Vida, or a sibling at all.

'Does this happen often?' I ask.

'Not often, no. But not everyone is a good candidate for IVF. Some women just don't respond to the medication.'

And so my IVF 'journey' ends. I am briefly crushed by its abrupt finish, but I surprise myself with a measured response: it feels something like relief.

I go to the clinic the following day for a blood test, to check that nothing has changed overnight. It hasn't; my progesterone still plods along, my ovaries clearly unwilling to be hassled into anything. I step out into the icy air outside, head straight to a café and order a double-shot coffee, my first caffeine in a week. And for the first time in a while, I feel I can be kind to myself – this isn't my fault. Much as I'd treated the IVF as a project, something within my control, of course it wasn't. I went into it with a womb and a budget, but they weren't enough.

If Vida ever needs a transplant, we'll have to put our faith in an unrelated donor. Either that or, who knows, maybe we'll be one of the couples to conceive a matched sibling baby naturally. I wouldn't have dared to take the risk of doing either before, but now I have the permission to steel myself, to help my daughter through whatever means and to make new life the way I know how. I am running towards life – my children's, and my own.

February arrives, Vida's birthday month. It has been looming, a reminder of the chasm between now and twelve months ago. I remember how we gazed at the swaddled mass of our daughter on the first night, unaware of what lay ahead; of those first eleven weeks and five days, when we had screeched through parenthood like nails on a blackboard, the discord intensifying as her blood count dropped.

Once Vida's first birthday has passed, I anticipate other anniversaries: my own birthday in April, when last year we went out for lunch and pretended that drinking wine and eating fried food with a mercilessly crying baby was no big deal; 13 May, that awful first day at Lewisham; 4 July, diagnosis; 18 July, the first clinic with Josu. Dates are beacons, accenting the days so that time can't simply plod forward to make its healing buffer. Dates arrest, they don't let me get too comfortable. They also come hand in hand with environmental triggers – sometimes happy ones, like mimosa blossom and bright, freezing February days around the time of Vida's birth, but also the blue skies of summer, when everyone comes out – and, last year, when I went in.

I am not alone in finding that anniversaries set something off in me. I've read a bit about the anniversary reaction; apparently certain responses to anniversaries associated with a trauma can be considered symptomatic of PTSD. Perhaps my dread would better stand to reason were it stemming from a bereavement, significant dates a reminder of the distance between you and your loved one; the pressure, maybe, to 'move on', most likely before you are ready. But we have all emerged from our trauma alive, and I have learnt not to take this for granted. I do not want DBA to taint a birthday that, if anything, should be an even bigger celebration than it would otherwise. Vida isn't just here; she is flourishing.

She is due a transfusion in her birthday week and I book it for the day before, determined for her to feel her best for the big day. We can't party without haemoglobin. In the afternoon on Snow Fox, the whole nursing team surprise her with a Black Forest gateau. (It later emerges that this is not laid on by the hospital but something that the staff personally club together and make happen.) I still have the video; there must be fifteen of them singing. She watches them from her buggy – singing to *her!* – with a look of confused wonder, liking it, but a little too shocked to smile. The last time we heard anyone singing 'Happy Birthday' in hospital was in A & E last May, the day of that first admission, a day when revelry felt like another country. But not today.

On her birthday itself, she takes no pleasure in my efforts to enhance her breakfast. She doesn't notice the cream in her porridge, and she isn't interested in the orange juice I have squeezed. But she loves the helium dog balloons sent by family friends, which pop out of an enormous box and are the highlight not just of the day but the entire month, until their heads start to flop. Lauren has sent a tea set with two dolls embroidered with our daughters' names; Zoe sends a set of wooden Winnie-the-Pooh skittles. It is a coincidence that Vida homes in on the presents sent by our new DBA friends, but it feels poignant. They are instant favourites and, years on at the time of writing, still are.

It's a happy day. Freddie skips work and we go to the church music group, followed by a lunch of sushi where Vida refuses all offers of our food but wolfs down a pouch of shop-bought purée. The heresy! But at least she is eating, and I am too. Food is tasting good again.

At the weekend, the day before my maternity leave ends, we have a party at Louise's house. We know it is significant to do this, but not quite *how* so. There are rumblings in the news about a virus that has swept across China, worlds away from West Hampstead. This, however, will turn out to be the last time we see our family and friends before Covid-19 reaches the UK, pushing the country into its first lockdown. For a second year running, Vida's birthday becomes a marker of blissful ignorance to what will ensue – this time, not to anything so niche as DBA.

For now, though, we eat cake. A rather splendid one: a four-tiered vanilla and buttercream cake with a golden carousel decoration that declares 'Happy 1st Birthday, Vida!' Boo has made cupcakes that we dot around it, each crowned with a golden carousel horse. After we have sung, Freddie says a few words, thanking people for their support during the last year. I had imagined crying when this happened, all my tension and sadness and resentment of the healthy children in the room surfaced by public acknowledgement. But I don't. The photographs of that day tell a tale of a family of three surrounded by people who care about them. Which is exactly what we are.

Until the day my maternity leave ends, my return to work has been a mirage – not anathema exactly, just difficult to believe. I am so altered. I must look much the same to my colleagues; little do they know the change that's occurred inside this skin. All returning mothers probably feel a degree of this, but I suspect for me it is less the fact of becoming a mother than the sense of having survived something unusually hard.

It has seemed ludicrous to me that I could just pick up where I left off at the *Guardian*, commissioning recipes for the weekend food section – deadlines, trend-spotting, proofreading. How many grams of spice in a teaspoon? Conventional or fan oven? Don't forget that soy contains gluten! And honey isn't vegan! I wonder how I will force myself to care again.

I have dedicated myself to food journalism for the last ten years and am lucky to have a job in a tiny and desirable industry. Exercising choice about what you eat and how you cook is more elitist than it should be, not least because there are so many tiers of quality to even the most basic of foodstuffs: bread, milk, vegetables. I am aware of how important the *Guardian*'s food section is to selling print copies of the Saturday paper – the pictures of pies and puds that are splashed across the masthead promoting the consumption of a lifestyle idea as much as food itself – and no area of publishing has boomed quite like the cookery sector in recent decades. Cookbooks and magazines don't just contain the instructions to make a tasty meal. With their glossy food styling, impeccably chosen props and, often, jaw-dropping kitchen interiors, they sell us the life we want. It's aspiration at its most delicious.

Before Vida, this was my world. I make no bones about how image-conscious I had become. I knew how I liked things, be they food and drink, what I wore, and my surroundings because I was – I am – privileged. The idea of 'me' was neatly expressed by my Instagram grid, which gave away what I was happy for people to see and think about my life. I knew I was much more than an assemblage of tiles – photos I'd pored over taking, styling, posting – but I also believed that version of it. It was truthful insofar as any one-dimensional story is. When I added another photo of my new baby's feet next to a plate of Marmite on toast in my lap in February 2019, it was merely another piece of scaffolding in the delicate construction of my sort-of life. When Vida became seriously ill, the structure tumbled spectacularly.

I'd been dreading this moment, but as I walk back into the *Guardian* offices, sit down at my desk and see my colleagues together for the first time in a year, it feels comfortable. They know something unexpected happened on my maternity leave, but not the extent of it. I throw myself back into edits – un-splitting infinitives, rejigging, reshaping. (If only I could edit genetic code this easily.) Commissioning again feels good too, cherry-picking dishes from lists of sumptuous ideas that celebrate seasons and store cupboards, curating each issue so that the recipes complement one another, or at least cover different ground. I work hard at making and commanding a tidy schedule.

On the days I am here, there are moments when it feels like the past. I left for and return from maternity leave in February, the month of forced rhubarb and Valentine's desserts! But I'm also back in my old habit scouring Mumsnet forums for signs that I might be pregnant. I had expected to come back to work in the throes of IVF but have instead returned to the slog of trying to conceive naturally. We're both hoping it won't be as testing as last time.

At the same time, the news is full of the spread of coronavirus. Since Vida's party, Freddie has been wary of going to any of the other NCT birthday gatherings. He also moots stocking up on food. In fact, he does this several times and we laugh at him – not for his anxiety (in that he will be vindicated), but for his choice of 'essential' items (the likes of Parma ham and blood-orange juice).

Initially, I pay little notice to the virus and apply an *it'll-probably-be-alright* mentality. It feels far away, but the situation intensifies quickly. Public transport empties, supermarket shelves are cleared of dry goods, hands chap from washing and sanitising. Coronavirus becomes Covid–19 becomes simply Covid; we start to hear of deaths, not just in the headlines but in text messages, relatives of people we know and care about; on 11 March 2020 it officially becomes a pandemic.

These are frightening times, not least because so little is known about Covid – and, for us, how it might affect people with blood disorders like DBA. I become aware that other families are choosing to withdraw their DBA children from childcare or school, isolating from mainstream society and becoming registered on the clinically extremely vulnerable list. It is at this point that I decide to work from home, two weeks before the whole country is ordered to do so. Key workers, like the doctors and nurses at Snow Fox and St Mary's PHDU (Paediatric Haematology Day Unit), have to continue to go in, of course. And we too must keep going to hospital, which is largely touted as the riskiest place to be, swarming with airborne particles coughed up by the nation's sickest. But when you're going in for life-saving treatment, the threat of other things retreats; we have no choice.

My own response to the arrival of Covid is different from Freddie's. More than once, we disagree about this, he flummoxed by my sanguine approach to global crisis. It's not that the virus doesn't worry me, or that I don't feel the need to be cautious – I've taken to wearing face masks and to washing my hands rigorously for the suggested twenty seconds. And I certainly know better than to assume that I or my family are immune to illness. Evidence is emerging about the risk to different demographics and suggests that Freddie, Vida and I are probably relatively safe (DBA notwithstanding), but that – given their ages and pre-existing health conditions – our parents might not be. I *do* worry about them getting ill, about us giving Covid to them. But my worry takes the form of minimising risk without trying to control the uncontrollable.

Do I feel cushioned, somehow, from this new fear, having experienced another kind so sharply and recently? Not exactly. And it's not that I live in denial about Covid's threat, either: I know Freddie, who has anti-bac spray by the door and makes us change and shower as soon as we've come in from being outdoors, is right to be worried. The panic surrounding me, however, somehow undoes my own, neutralising some of the lonely agitation I have felt over so much of the last year.

A month or so into lockdown, Louise will comment that a number of her psychotherapy patients are doing better during the pandemic than before. Speaking on Louis Theroux's lockdown podcast, the journalist Jon Ronson alludes to something comparable, saying, 'There's a weird phenomenon, which I'm sure you've noticed . . . that people with anxiety disorders are coping especially well in this situation.' He continues: 'When coronavirus started, like a lot of people with anxiety, I found myself very, like, calm and focused. It's like: OK I've been preparing for this my whole life, so this is what I have to do.' In my case, I haven't so much been waiting for a catastrophe; the catastrophe has already happened. Covid is a concern shared by everyone and it is a welcome change from wrangling medical uncertainty and a vulnerable child alone with Freddie.

While hovering on Facebook, I start to notice DBA parents worrying about blood supplies. Lockdown measures are extreme; if people are only leaving their homes to get essential groceries, or for their daily exercise, blood donations are sure to drop. And donors can be forgiven for fearing it –

getting on public transport to give blood in a medical facility sits at odds with the government's advice to stay at home. While I am confident that, given our London base and Vida's common blood type, she will continue to get the blood she needs, it has been mooted that some transfusion-dependent children might have to be transfused less often. Moving from every three weeks to every four would not be good for Vida, who we have seen becomes symptomatic just before her three-weekly transfusion, refusing mouthfuls of even the foods she likes most and turning her head away from her bottle of warm milk at bedtime before she has finished it.

I make an Instagram post on a whim. I haven't used the app for ten months. I explain to my following that I've taken a break, that this is my daughter, that she has this condition which makes her dependent on blood transfusions – and to please give blood. I become choked up as soon as it's done. This is a first. Owning things so publicly is ultimately positive – I don't want Vida's condition to be shrouded in secrecy simply because it is invisible, and I believe that claiming it will both empower her and normalise it, just another kind of difference in a world full of different people. I look at the post as an outsider might – does it invite pity? Am I compounding the viewer's sense – a sense which I might once have had – that things like this didn't happen to them, that despite the feeling of proximity that social media brings, my circumstances are so very far from their own?

The response amazes me, though. It's an explosion of support. Lots of people tell me they are regular blood donors, others resolve to sign up. Lots more send love. I receive a few private messages from people who have had similar experiences – of caring for unwell children, or who have been ill themselves, describing the strain that it put on their mental health. There are even one or two who have or know a child with DBA. Conversations start, relationships are forged. With every kind comment, I am reeled back into an online community which I'd found so toxic ten months before.

Rachel Cusk wrote that childcare manuals were 'the emblem of the new mother's psychic loneliness' and I had certainly felt this on leafing through the likes of *What to Expect* and *Your Baby Week-by-Week* in between failed naps and curtailed feeds. With their presumptions of normality, their advice was alienatingly generic, a reminder of everything that wasn't going 'right' or 'well' or 'to plan'. But, I imagined, if your baby did everything quite literally by the book, these same books would be so confidence-boosting, so feel-good. Social media intensifies this effect: how lonely all that scrolling had made me feel, how dangerous the cumulative effect of all those filtered, seemingly picture-perfect lives.

Yet how comforting now, to know from people who had once approved of my own filtered life with their 'likes' and emojis and comments, that they see me in this new place and can tell me that I'm not alone. There is value in that, too.

I was born in St George's Hospital, Tooting, in 1985 and I grew up in West Norwood, a once unremarkable suburb to the south of the city known for having one of London's 'Magnificent Seven' cemeteries. West Norwood is now another London enclave with coffee and sourdough pizza, which would have been hard to imagine during my childhood. Our house was opposite a Victorian orphanage-turned-council building; now, at the time of writing, it's a well-respected primary school. On our street corner there was a massage parlour called Sparkles with a neon sign and windows painted in pink; today it is a development of flats, which I suspect command eyebrow-raising prices.

Save for my university years in Leeds and my time in America, I have always lived in London. I shifted around flats in the south – Brixton, Clapham, Balham – until I moved in with Freddie and Louise in the north-west. He and I then settled (or so we thought) in Lewisham. I have thirty-four years of memories mapped across this city. So many of its contours are overlaid for me with past events, distant feelings. Karl Marx reportedly said that 'Men can see nothing around them that is not their own image; everything speaks to them of themselves. Their very landscape is alive.' I didn't think London could feel any more alive to me, because I had lived so much and so fully here. It was, I thought, as familiar as a place could be.

But the last year has given me a new perspective on the place I was born. Areas are no longer defined by museums, or restaurants, or pubs, but by hospitals. We have been to nine in London this year, all for different things according to their specialisms and/or locations – Lewisham, to give birth; King's, for the tongue-tie clinic; the Whittington, for A & E; Guy's, for genetics and psychiatry; the Brompton, for paediatric cardiology; St Thomas' and the Evelina, for paediatric haematology; St Mary's, for specialist haematology; the Royal Free, for pre-IVF bloods; St George's, for our PREGCARE samples. And that's not counting all the health centres for routine medical care – GP appointments, getting Vida weighed and vaccinated. Medical centres are now major points of interest in the algorithm of my Google Maps.

We navigate the place differently too, often driving across town at rush hour, which I'd spent a lifetime trying to avoid. I have been grateful for the car, though, which on many occasions has ferried us to appointments and shielded me from minor interactions, like asking for help with the buggy at the bottom of a Tube-station staircase. From inside the car, I can, with cool detachment, look upon the city at its loveliest angles. The novelty of driving down Constitution Hill, seeing Buckingham Palace and the mounted guards, the snowdrops and the joggers, and absorbing it all without the pressure of a taxi meter ticking upwards will perhaps never wear off.

Oddly though, despite trying to avoid other people, I don't think I've ever felt more a part of London than I do now. With our new dependence on its services has come a different sense of belonging. This may result from the tyranny of having no choice, but I find myself proud to know my city in this way. I am learning what it feels like to be invested – not just in principle, but in practice. Sometimes at the Evelina, while Vida's transfusion runs, I will go to the parents' kitchen to make a cup of tea and look over the river at the Houses of Parliament. I think how acutely the people on this ward feel some of the decisions made over there.

Sometimes events of the last year catch up with me. Walking from one room to another, say, the world spins and stops me in my tracks. Vertigo. I have come to recognise this as disbelief, which I feel with my whole body. *Five to seven babies with DBA in a million live births. Bone marrow register. Genetic disorder.* Is it definitely not a dream? The writer Masha Gessen calls these 'moments that ... overwhelm [the] imagination with their absurdity'.

Once they're a year old, DBA patients have some of the interventions that make the road ahead look a bit clearer. Most often, this starts with a biopsy to establish the condition of the bone marrow. The most significant measure for this is 'cellularity', which indicates what percentage of the bone marrow is productive. Once Josu has a gauge of this, the plan is usually to start a month-long course of high-dose steroids in the hope that they will kickstart red-cell production.

Already in the news there are noises about routine hospital procedures being cancelled or indefinitely postponed, to prioritise the many thousands of Covid-19 patients. Vida's biopsy is booked for my second week back at work, just after her first birthday, and while it feels odd to take time off so soon, I want to make sure it happens promptly.

We are required at a pre-op appointment two days before, to check she is well and to consent to the various risks associated with a general anaesthetic. This is our first experience of signing up to a risk in Vida's interests, of choosing the least bad option in an un-ideal scenario. It won't be the last time; in years to come, I will learn to shrug off the fearsome possibilities intrinsic to these things – anaesthetics, transfusions and medications. They will become almost as mundane as brushing my teeth, some of the things we do to keep our family intact. But this first time, I feel that spin of disbelief as I make my inaugural scribble on a consent form, my senses overwhelmed by the absurdity of it all.

I wasn't prepared for the sight of my daughter in a hospital gown. It's covered in faded teddy bears and she looks tiny and shapeless in it, only the faint line of her nappy visible underneath. She sits perkily in my arms as we walk into the theatre, unaware of what is about to happen. I wasn't prepared for the next bit, either, when she is put to sleep for the operation.

While I cradle her, the anaesthetist holds a child-sized mask near her face, then over it. She wriggles, worried, then surrenders, taut muscles submitting to the gas. The play therapist blows bubbles until her eyes close. I rest a hand on her tummy, feel it rise and fall steadily.

'OK, give her a kiss,' says the anaesthetist. I do, and Freddie leans over us to do the same. I lay her on the bed. Her face is peaceful, like best china – pristine, breakable. The idea of leaving her now is obscene, a wilful violation of my protector role. When I turn around, Freddie is there. He clutches the knitted tiger he bought her in Lewisham, eyes full, cheeks wet. I wasn't prepared for any of this.

A bone-marrow biopsy is surprisingly straightforward. Once the patient is asleep, a needle is inserted into the back of the hip and an aspiration of marrow is taken.

It won't take long, we are told, and are encouraged to pop out for a walk. St Mary's Hospital is just over Paddington Basin from Paddington station. In months to come, Vida will be delighted by all the nods to the eponymous bear en route to see Josu; as we walk along the canal – the Westway roaring behind us – she will look forward to the blue, 'life-size', felt-covered Paddington mannequin beside the colourful barge. He doffs his hat. I have a photo of her, aged two and a half, gleeful in her buggy beside him. Little perks like this are important on our hospital days – when we go to the Evelina, we always pay a visit to the 'Bah-Bah Wheel' (the Great Big Wheel, or London Eye), which thrills her in winter in particular, when it is lit up in pink against the dark night sky.

Freddie and I head out for a coffee, and almost as soon as we step back onto the ward, it is time to find Vida in the recovery room. She is discombobulated and crying – I am uncomfortable about not being there when she woke up but was told this was unavoidable. I think she has only just come to when I arrive, armed with warm milk and a Philadelphia sandwich. She guzzles both, ravenous after being nil by mouth since last night.

She is left with a red speck where the aspirate was taken, which will harden into scar tissue, a chapter in the story her body will tell. The happier outcome of general anaesthetic has been the insertion of a cannula without Vida's noticing. We have decided to combine today's admission with a blood transfusion – it is a plus for the cannula to have gone in without the usual three-weekly tussle and tears.

When the country goes into its first Covid lockdown, Freddie, Louise and I are all suddenly at home, on a hamster wheel of work, childcare and *PE with Joe* workouts. Well, the others do Joe Wicks. I attempt some jogs around the block, but chasing around after my just-walking now toddler is a workout enough. She's very gung-ho, flinging herself between sofas before she buckles. No sooner has she started toddling when the climbing begins.

As Vida is on the move, and Louise's work still requires a quiet house, we have to shut ourselves in the living room. It is a good thing that we don't yet know how long this lockdown will last – confined to one room, we all quickly get cabin fever. Whenever the door opens, Vida cries out desperately. Her world is shrinking right when it should expand.

We meet Josu for clinic online, a first. The NHS is shifting as many appointments online as possible to minimise the risk of exposure to Covid. Vida's biopsy results are disappointing. She is hypocellular, which means that less than 30 per cent of her bone marrow is producing cells. Josu tells us that it could improve, but that this is unusual. All steroid trials are being postponed – children on the high dose are immunosuppressed, and no doctor wants to take undue risks right now. At this stage, little is known about Covid and its effect on people with blood disorders. We obviously want to keep Vida safe, but this is all still a blow to me – a spanner in the works of progress. Instead of starting steroids, Josu says we should begin Exjade, the oral chelation medicine, because the iron levels in her blood are high.

What did I expect to hear? With every face-to-face with her doctor, a part of me still hopes, I think, that they'll have got this diagnosis wrong. That it isn't as they thought, that there's no DBA here; what novelist Maggie O'Farrell described as 'some frail, furled part of [her] that is hoping there has been a mistake'.

After the appointment, I go to the park and call my mum, distraught. Ernie runs over to the magpies ahead of me, disbanding their peaceful breakfast. There is a well-trodden path through these fields that, like every winter before it, has become a bog, its edges only just starting to harden. I squelch through, covering my legs in soupy mud; I have an urge to feel the chaos of things physically. To wear the mess in my mind. Joggers and dog walkers, eagerly taking their exercise for the day before locking down again at home, pass me, undoubtedly see my wet face, hair caught in my streaming nose, my short, shallow breaths. I don't care. I need this cry. I am due a Shakespearean moment.

This won't be the last time that I am thrown by news from Vida's medical team. I had adjusted to our new routine, one which had so horrified me eight months ago, and I was on my way to accepting how our life was going to be. But today I have been reminded of the seriousness of things, undoing a bit of the normalising I'd been working on so hard.

This virus has come along and rerouted us. In time, I will feel grateful that Vida started iron chelation sooner than expected and that her steroids were delayed, allowing her a little more time to grow and thrive. But none of that is the point right now. I have been clinging to the few knowns available in our new DBA life: that Vida would start steroids at one year old had seemed a reliable fact. Once again, I am derailed by our script, which is less a script than a constant improvisation. You couldn't write any of it.

I have never been a spreadsheet person and am faithful to my paper diary, which I am poor at updating and often forget to carry with me. But I take to a menstrual tracking app like a pro, inputting everything from periods to whether I've had a positive ovulation-test stick. You'd have thought I would know better than to think I could control the course of biology by now. But having a project helps.

It's an incongruously beautiful spring. Every morning, I take Ernie to Hampstead Heath under a glorious sky – I can't remember a brighter, greener April. Nature is marching us all forward, reminding us that it is more than the spheres and spikes of coronavirus: it is the sun piercing a glowing canopy, voluptuous clouds and quick showers; cow parsley, frogspawn and silt; mud, peat and weeds.

Vida's breakfast is always porridge with nutmeg, mashed banana, peanut butter. Now, though, her first few mouthfuls are sprinkled with a crushed-up pill. She has never eaten with much gusto, always sensitive to changes in taste or texture, so we had wondered how Exjade would go down. But it slips in just fine.

I keep being surprised in ways like this – by Vida, by myself. I am enjoying cooking again, my appetite sparked by the recipes we are featuring in the magazine. Now more than ever, cooking feels transportive. My friend and columnist, Rachel Roddy, whose writing always makes me want to cook, has done a new take on Roman beans and greens, which makes the kitchen feel both like home and somewhere else – oil, onion and garlic conspiring with pulse and vegetable in alchemical ways. Even Vida can't resist.

The hospital has introduced a single-parent policy for Covid infection control. There was always going to be a time when I would have to bring Vida for a transfusion on my own, but this is sooner than expected. We are filled with trepidation at the prospect. In the past, on days when Freddie had to work, one of our parents would join me. Now only the most essential people can come.

Vida is too young to sit quietly in front of the television, nor is she interested in the play therapist and her box of toy dinosaurs. She is a busy fourteen-month-old unwillingly tethered to a bag of blood, fidgeting on her mum's lap. Transfusion days are becoming more physical; the cannula is always a battle, but now that she no longer breastfeeds, there's no way to make sure she sleeps for some of it. If she does, she is usually disturbed by a nurse coming to do a set of observations. Three and a half hours, the current typical length of a transfusion, feels very long. The blood travels so slowly through the line that you can't even see it moving; a drip falls from the bag into a test tube that leads to the line every two or three seconds, the only indication of movement. I buy my muscles some time out and give Vida a bottle of milk, feeling her body relax against mine – a moment's repose.

I take out my phone. In the old days, when I was procrastinating at work, I would open a new window in my web browser, often typing in *faceb*— before catching myself in the act. Now, my menstrual tracking app has replaced Facebook as my tech twitch of choice, the lives lived by others far less appealing than the potential for life within me. Technology is perverse – its notifications, flashing smiley faces and acronym-packed forums offering an illusion of control. I read about SMEP, the Sperm Meets Egg Plan, which I study seriously, ignoring the fact that it's really just the advice to shag every other day. SMEP suggests structure, and structure suggests something to follow that leads to success – the paint-by-numbers of conception.

This transfusion, number seventeen, eventually ends and Vida is unplugged, unwrapped, the teddy bears unstuck with an adhesive-remover. The cannula is taken out, and I am asked to hold a bunny tail of cotton wool tightly over the site to stem the flow of blood while it clots. My jeans are covered in a rubble of squashed cheese that escaped from a sandwich.

Before we go, I wheel the buggy into the disabled loo on Snow Fox and notice I have bled. My heart sinks as I realise another month of trying to conceive has bitten the dust.

—

The specialist nurse at St Mary's has been encouraging me to apply for Disability Living Allowance (DLA) on Vida's behalf. I have resisted doing so for months: filling out paperwork to prove her body's limitations, and the challenges we face, feels counterintuitive to the process of acceptance and minimising that I have been through. It is an exercise in highlighting, with as much detail as possible, how much more help Vida needs than a typically healthy child. Doing so threatens to draw me backwards.

However, as I keep reminding myself, this isn't about me and my fragility – or it can't be any more. Given how disproportionately difficult and expensive life can be for many families dealing with a disability, Disability Living Allowance is a meagre sum, even at the highest level. But there are good reasons to apply, aside from the money; if we are successful with our application, Vida will gain early entitlement to attend an excellent nearby nursery for free. It's worth it.

I brace myself and start filling in the form. To my surprise, it feels not unlike writing the beginnings of that Instagram post, and somehow it puts air in my lungs. I put our trajectory of parenthood into my own words and make a strong statement of the hard facts. In retelling it, I feel less of the sadness. It will take several appeals and a tribunal before Vida is eventually granted DLA (at the lowest level) a year later, but the process of getting there was as important as the outcome.

I wait for my period to start in earnest. It doesn't. I don't think too much of this at first. In the past I have been through many months of trying to get pregnant, convincing myself that spots of blood aren't menstrual but, in fact, 'implantation bleeding', the name for when a newly fertilised egg burrows into the uterine wall and causes a small amount of blood loss. I've read about it and it seems to be a thing, but I know better than to hope it might be the case for me.

Still, I wake up five days after the transfusion and still no period. Outside, it is a bright morning and the trees are irrepressibly green. Before Vida wakes up, I take a pregnancy test on a whim and am met with two strong, dark blue lines.

I blink and they are still there.

I lean back on the cistern for a moment, alone with the news. I feel as much raw delight as I did in Cornwall on that similarly bright morning twenty-one months ago, if a little more knowing than I was then. *Here we go*, I think. Also, *hello*, to whoever is in there. Other thoughts simmer, of course, how could they not? But I won't let them take this moment from me, as I have on so many occasions in the last year.

In a few weeks, it will be a year since Vida's first admission to Lewisham. Things move forward, inexorably. Chapters we wrote with our genes are publishing. We are here – three, nearly four, of us. And I will go to the park in the next hour and I know I will see my pair of magpies digging for worms, as they do every morning. Two for joy.

Blood is an international currency. We all spend it. Our bodies work hard to earn it. It's a constant economy of breath, energy and protein.

I knew that blood was vital before I had Vida, but only

in abstract; it was like crypto, more of an idea than a thing of material value – a kind of precious mystery. For Goethe, it was 'a very special juice'; for Joyce Carol Oates, 'blood is memory without language'; Jim Morrison described it as 'the rose of mysterious union'. An enigmatic holder of clues, of history, its appearance a sign both of life and of death. I thought little of all this before. Blood had been periods and torn cuticles; a bitten lip, perhaps, or the slip of a kitchen knife. Like oxygen and life itself, I took blood for granted.

Now I notice it everywhere – vivid, unmissable. In traffic, NHS Blood and Transplant motorbikes weave around other vehicles, transporting bags of it around the city. In faces, flushed. On plates, mingling with fat from just-cooked meat. On menus, bone marrow, blood sausage, black pudding. In words, it is emotive and often throwaway: warming in passion, boiling in anger, running cold in fear, curdling when we are shaken. Blood suggests alliance, bonded by blood, but also enmity: 'blood will have blood', as Macbeth had it.

Belonging, family, loyalty. Pain, suffering, sacrifice. One's very essence, to be alive, to die. It is a fact that Vida's A+ blood derives from my O+ and Freddie's A– ; figuratively, we share blood, too: we are blood relatives. 'Blood is thicker than water,' goes the saying, and I don't always agree, but I do know that the blood I share with Vida is thicker than anything I've ever known.

The summer of 2020 is a strangely happy one. Strangely, because I am sick as a dog and events in the outside world seem apocalyptic. Chaos reigns in the headlines – Covid's rising death toll, negligent leadership, the tragic murder of George Floyd in Minneapolis and the following civil rights protests across much of the world. As unsafe as I have felt in the last year, I see now, tucked away in lockdown with Vida, how safe I really am. Enjoying my relative comfort in this moment feels important, an act of gratitude.

We eat very well, despite having some teething problems with the major supermarkets around Vida's clinically vulnerable status. They seem resistant to putting us on the high-priority list for food deliveries, probably because DBA is so little known. So instead, we buy a lot of our food from wholesalers, which have been forced to pivot by restaurant closures. At night, once Vida is asleep, I eat summer fruits in bed. The first baby I grew demanded grapefruit; the second is here for the peaches and nectarines, cherries and apricots.

Tastes, words, sounds and images, which all seemed so meaningless last summer, are newly delicious. Sometimes they astound me. I watch Michaela Coel's masterpiece, *I May Destroy You*, and the adaptation of Sally Rooney's *Normal People*, and I read Bernadine Evaristo's *Girl, Woman, Other* and Brit Bennett's *The Vanishing Half*. Freddie buys a cello and starts online lessons; I hear him swiping and riffing and singing in the room next door, and the result is the makings of his band's first album; I make Alison Roman's Tiny, Salty, Chócolaty Cookies and my Cretan chef friend Marianna's deep-fried courgette fritters with feta, mint and oregano, and eat them alongside bulging, ripe tomatoes. I feel amazed by human industry, by the power to make and to consume, and by how much it all helps.

Freddie is convinced the baby is another girl, probably, he says, because having a girl is what he already knows. I am on the fence.

We bandy names about – the girls' names we hadn't used the first time around, and some new ones that go well with Vida. We find it harder to agree on one for a boy. Somehow, girls' names allow for more creative licence. We ponder whether this is patriarchy working in its insidious way.

There are, of course, strong arguments for finding a gender-neutral name, but this isn't easy with all the criteria that need to be met. These include that it needs to work with an exceptionally long surname and string of middle names, including a bird species, a convention on my mum's side of the family, and that, as we have calculated that the baby will definitely be born in December, we want something a bit festive. Yes, we are that cheesy.

Vida is no longer the only patient of St Thomas' hospital in our family. I have self-referred to their maternity service: I find the hospital's size and central location reassuring, but more importantly, it is somewhere that attracts leading medics. Since Vida's diagnosis, I have come across plenty of doctors who have never heard of DBA and I want to be under the care of a place not only familiar with the condition, but familiar with my family.

Covid rules stop Freddie from joining me at the early antenatal appointments. My disappointment about this gives way to a kind of perverse relief. I suspect he feels the same. We have been through a lot together, and our anxieties have a tendency to cross-pollinate. I feel protective both of our baby, who I would like to spare any undue shots of cortisol, but also of Freddie. I am fine with keeping my triggering questions for the experts.

I'm immediately assigned a lovely midwife who specialises in maternal mental health, and who stays in regular contact throughout my pregnancy. In the first few months, I am also referred to a foetal medicine consultant, who checks the growing baby for anomalies with his battery of tricks: Dopplers, sonography, ranges. The consultant loves the *Guardian*'s food offering and happens to have read the article I wrote about Vida's diagnosis. We bond over Ottolenghi and foetal health.

Together we weigh up the advantages of prenatal testing. After all that has happened, I am keen to know if our new baby might have DBA. While we know the chances are low, anything seems possible.

Screening a growing foetus for health conditions is a thorny issue. If a baby is positive for anything, I firmly believe that the parents' decision is personal, private, and should be unfettered by theoretical ethics. We haven't got as far as discussing what we would do in the event of Vida's sibling also having an illness; we just want to be prepared for any eventuality. I have learnt that when it comes to babies, I don't want surprises.

When I am ten weeks pregnant, I have the private Harmony test to look for chromosomal abnormalities. We find the baby has none that they can test for. We also find out that we are having a boy. He is due to join us just after Christmas. He becomes less abstract with every passing day and, not to get too Pinocchio about it, more of a real boy. There is beauty in the knowledge of what's to come, yet there's also the worry that he may have DBA and that if he does, he will likely have to go through all that Vida does.

So, we have two options: chorionic villus sampling (CVS), where a few cells from the placenta are tested at around eleven weeks of pregnancy, or amniocentesis, where a small amount of the amniotic fluid around the foetus is taken via a tiny needle at about sixteen weeks. Both are invasive, neither is without risk. We plan for CVS because this way we'll know sooner, but on the two days we try, the consultant is concerned that there are too many blood vessels surrounding my placenta and that it wouldn't be safe. So we wait to do amniocentesis. And at sixteen weeks, I see my baby's profile onscreen – his nose more defined than three weeks ago, his tiny hand waving, his alien legs wriggling – and I take pause.

'You do realise there's a higher chance of you miscarrying as a result of amniocentesis than of this baby having Diamond-Blackfan, don't you?' says the consultant.

I do realise this. One in a hundred amnioceteses harm the baby. Five to seven in a million live births have DBA. And if this baby has DBA – well, we already have a joyful child with the condition whose life is largely good.

It suddenly feels like a no-brainer. I leave without doing the test, but I do request to keep this consultant for the rest of the pregnancy. We know each other a bit now.

Save for the remarkable din of the pandemic, most of my pregnancy has been unremarkable. True to form, my sickness subsides at fourteen weeks. I get sciatica in a major way and can only crawl up the stairs by the time I reach thirty-four weeks. Carrying Vida has become very difficult, not least because she is now twenty months old.

The risk of catching Covid while pregnant means Freddie has taken sole charge of transfusion days, minimising my contact with hospitals – I only visit the hospital for foetal medicine scans. Everything else takes place virtually. Pregnant women all over the country must give birth on their own, without their partners. We stay hopeful that by the time our boy is born, those restrictions might have relaxed.

I had not felt unduly worried about catching Covid myself, even as a pregnant woman. I'm sure that DBA had a part to play in my ease; on some level, I felt I'd already been through the mill, and I didn't think my catching Covid could be a worse ordeal. I was, however, *very* worried about Vida getting it and so, much as I accepted the limits of my control over this bug, I had diligently taken precautions and shielded as much as possible.

I have no idea where or how I caught it. I went to so few places in those months. But I remember the first cough, on the way home from a thirty-six-week scan. It was just one cough, nothing unusual. But somehow I just knew.

After a night of fitful sleep, I drive to a mobile testing unit in a Brixton car park to take a test. I hadn't had the results at bedtime, but in the darkness I reach for my phone – the nervous twitch of our time – and embark on an insomnia scroll. And there it is, before I can open Instagram or the news, an email with the result. Positive.

The next six days pass in a fog of sweaty pyjamas and breathlessness. All three of us have tested positive for Covid, but Freddie and Vida are not symptomatic, so far. I quickly find standing up intolerable, am utterly dysfunctional, periodically shivering my way to the bathroom on all fours.

Freddie becomes sole carer for Vida, whose energy has not waned. He buys countless stickers, Amazon parcels of crafts and kinetic sand. My cousin Will, Vida's godfather, makes her an Advent calendar of presents for a daily novelty: farm animals, chocolate buttons, stones from a Norfolk beach. There's also a lot of CBeebies. To be honest, she's mostly interested in pulling the stuffing out of our blocked chimney, climbing on the table, pulling cookbooks off the shelves. I join them downstairs every so often, witness Freddie's hollow eyes as he muddles through. I can see he has been crying; once he does so in my presence and I realise he really thinks I might die.

I wait Covid out under the duvet, convinced that I am scaling its peak before my inevitable return to good health. We have booked an elective caesarean in two weeks' time – on the winter solstice! I have been romantically attached to this date and I am determined to make it. As the days roll on, though, I feel no better. At intervals, Freddie appears in the bedroom with tea, toast and an oxygen saturation ('sats') monitor he bought online. We watch the numbers over a couple of days and see my heart rate climb and my sats drop. The baby swirls reassuringly every so often. I notice that he no longer feels like a part of me, like we are one thing; now my hugeness – *his* hugeness – feels like an obstruction to my getting the air I need to keep us both going.

It's on the Thursday, six days after my positive result, that my sats hit their lowest yet. Freddie comes into the bedroom holding Vida. She wriggles in his arms, wanting me and the various trinkets on the ledge behind our bed. I am the least lucid I have been. Freddie is exhausted – cheeks pink, eyes tiny. He clips the sats monitor onto my finger, which flashes red with 87 per cent. He tells me he doesn't trust that he can look after me now; we need to call an ambulance.

Our son was born that evening. By the time he had arrived, and we'd been restored to an isolation cubicle on the St Thomas' maternity ward, Freddie's relief was so great that he let me choose his name.

'Whatever you want to call him xxxx,' said the message. Even though the birth fell in between two consecutive, tightly spaced lockdowns, when the rules on partners attending births had relaxed, Freddie was not allowed to be there. We were both Covid positive, and in any case, he needed to look after Vida because nobody else could. (Our friends Grace and Raffi risked their health and their Christmas by moving in with Vida and Fred for a few days. When I eventually came home, it would be to a freezer full of sugar-cookie dough and ingredients neatly arranged in chic plastic crates. Grace, it was revealed, is a Marie Kondo–Martha Stewart hybrid dream woman.)

So we settled on Gabriel. We needed an angel. A reassuringly bright pink angel, born in the least celestial of circumstances. And yet, for all that I wouldn't have chosen about how he landed, it was peaceful. People are horrified when I tell them I had him in this way, especially after all we had been through following Vida's birth, but those hackneyed phrases 'you're in the best place' or 'in the right hands' were true. I felt deep trust for St Thomas' hospital, confident that they would deliver the baby and get me better, which they did.

He had been whipped out within eight hours of my being admitted through A & E in an ambulance. The obstetricians were clear: the baby was big and occupying space in my abdomen that my lungs needed to expand into. Over the course of those hours, I was put on oxygen through a nasal catheter, which remained there for nearly a week. I was hooked up to observation machines 24/7, cannulated and given pain relief through an IV. Something they did helped quickly because I remember asking for food and slowly devouring, relishing, a plasticky white-bread cheese sandwich, which tasted amazing. Consultants came in and out. I think we had a conversation about steroids, a course of dexamethasone, which was being trialled on Covid patients.

It seems wrong that I have now forgotten so many names of the doctors and nurses to whom I might owe my life, not to mention that of my boy. These people were my lifeblood for a week. I remember characters, though. The anaesthetist who, once her work with the epidural was done, insisted I hand her my phone so she could film the birth. It is a video full of white noise and suction sounds, a primal scream and accompanying coos; I can hear myself saying quietly to the baby, 'Hello.' There are folds of green sterile fabric and clear plastic framing my white, blood-flecked belly, from which a large head and long body are pulled through an improbably small hole. The lighting is harsh on him, but watching it back, there is a theatrical quality to it: a spotlight on the star of the show, a halo on an angel.

It is three weeks before my due date; like Vida, Gabriel was born just after I'd turned thirty-seven weeks. He is about seven and a half pounds, and so, if left to his own devices, would have grown to be a big baby in those final weeks. There is so much of the boy I know now in those early expressions, a person whose default mode is one of good cheer, but who feels injustice and discomfort deeply. I'm not sure there's any injustice or discomfort quite like being born by caesarean section, so the strained, grumpy look on his face as he comes out seems entirely reasonable. First thoughts: an earthy, wide, full-cheeked face like mine and, yes, Freddie's signature frown. He is delicious.

—

Gabriel and I are alone together for his first seven days. I revel in his every snuffle, every grunt; the full-body stretches, the deep yawns. There has been a lot to test my ability to take pleasure in things recently. I am away from my home and husband, my daughter and the dog; I am also very ill, and fearful about history repeating itself, but nothing can tarnish my delight in this baby. In him I take the purest pleasure.

Of course, I cannot help but wonder whether he'll be a stem-cell match for Vida. We'd gone to such lengths to engineer a sibling donor for her at the beginning of the year. We might have decided to shelve that project, but I'd reserved a small morsel of hope that a match might come along naturally.

When I have trouble sleeping in Gabriel's early months, I will sometimes think about my week with him in hospital. The thought of it is an antidote to the panic I often feel when I lie awake in the small hours worrying about not sleeping. Casting my mind back to the maternity unit at St Thomas' slows my racing heart; I feel safe in the memory of it.

While for Freddie my Covid admission and emergency caesarean were traumatic, for me they were a lifeline. In hospital I felt held by medical expertise and round-the-clock care. I struggle to get out of bed for days and have help with everything: nappy changes, pumping milk, night feeds. I have slept terribly with Covid, but they are doing all they can here to help me rest. Once or twice, I open my eyes in the middle of the night to the sight of a midwife softly feeding Gabriel expressed milk from a tiny bottle.

Freddie has it harder than I do, I think. As the days pass, I feel incredulous that we have a son who he hasn't met – I suspect Freddie won't believe it himself until he meets him. Covid did not hit him anything like as badly as me, but it's always harder to be the one left behind. Especially when you're isolating with a toddler. Children force you to stay present, but they also deny you an escape. Without much sleep, and without the telly and other distractions, he scrambles for reasons to believe things will be OK. Freddie is a lifelong agnostic, but I find out later that during this time he contacted the vicar who married us and asked for his prayers.

We receive regular deliveries in hospital. Bags full of granny pants and tracksuit bottoms for me, Christmassy sleepsuits and miniscule nappies for Gabriel; also photographs of Vida, Freddie and Ernie to put up in the room, get-well-soon and new-baby cards, button-down pyjamas to wear while feeding. People are generous. My team at the *Guardian* send boxes of Middle Eastern food; there are cupcakes for me and a hamper of festive bakes for the midwives from my pastry-chef friend, Claire.

It's funny to think of those newborn days in the whole scheme of parenting small children. There is an absolute focus on keeping someone alive and getting yourself through it in one piece. It is gentle, dewy, as yet unharried by navigating plans with children in tow, packing up clobber and hurrying between places. It is as though baby and mother are born together, embarking on a journey of learning and relearning the world.

Seven days after his birth, Gabriel and I are allowed home. I have made good progress and haven't needed oxygen support for a couple of days. Freddie arrives with the baby car seat. He's wearing his mustard suit and Chelsea boots (I don't think I'll ever not be charmed by the effort he makes for important hospital visits) but I can tell he is shell-shocked. He is moved but reticent in meeting the baby, as though he can't quite believe that something so harrowing as the last two weeks could have resulted in something – someone – so lovely.

We head down to the car park together, a walk we have done many times. It is surreal to do this without Vida, who I could burst at the prospect of seeing in approximately thirty-five minutes.

We had Christmas at home – an uncertain eventuality while I was in hospital – and it was both magical and a bit haunting. Vida took great delight in our little tree (much more delight, it has to be said, than in her new brother, who she mostly ignored) and was mesmerised by baubles, periodically nicking and hiding them. She loved *The Snowman*, although wailed at the ending. She discovered gingerbread men. It was a Christmas of delicious firsts for her, and she was palpably happy to have her family back together. Now that we were all testing negative, her grandparents were around to help and, with the baby safely installed and everyone alive, there was a mood of rather manic jollity. The ordeal was catching up with Freddie and he was very quiet, hiding in the kitchen with the turkey – a responsibility he takes seriously at the best of times.

Gabriel had jaundice, as many newborn babies do, but it put us on high alert, because Vida had also been jaundiced. As instructed, I fed him through it, supplementing breastmilk with bottles and studying his colour in the morning light. On Christmas Eve we called the Lewisham jaundice clinic. On Christmas Day, we noticed he was breathing quickly. On Boxing Day, unable to bear the fear we both felt and then amplified in one another, we took him to paediatric A & E at St Thomas'. After three nights and clear blood tests, Gabriel was discharged with no concerns from doctors. After this, something clicked and I, at least, was able to enjoy my second baby, which was easier in many respects, not least because he slept for chunks of up to five hours.

It was a strange few months, a winter hibernation enforced by lockdown. We lived the merry-go-round of meals and nappies, bathtimes and night feeds, and it felt as bog-standard as life with small children goes. Already a second child had taken the emphasis off Diamond-Blackfan, which felt less of a defining feature of parenthood to me, although doubtless a presence in the room. That was certainly the case until, sometime in January, I received a phone call from the geneticist at Guy's. I was getting dressed while Gabriel gurgled on my bed, propped up by a pillow. Freddie happened to be outside the room, heard me answer, and then the lift in my voice when she told me that Gabriel did not have Vida's DBA mutation. Before I had even hung up, Freddie was on his knees, sobbing. The unspoken fear we'd shared – as we studied our baby's complexion for signs of anaemia each day, or pulled down his lower eyelids to reveal their membranes – had lifted in an instant.

About a month later, when I was walking to the park with Gabriel strapped to me, I received an email, this time from our specialist nurse at St Mary's. We had spoken just the night before about when the results of another genetic test might come back, which would tell us whether Gabriel was a potential donor for Vida.

> Nurse: Gabriel's report came through while we were talking about it last night! He is a match for Vida, should a transplant be warranted in the future.
>
> Me: Omg this is totally amazing
>
> Nurse: Sure is!

For a while, we can enjoy the little things. Playgrounds and soft plays, mud kitchens and bedtime stories. Hoping to set up a good sleep regime, I read the same book to Gabriel every night before I switch off the light, *Kissed by the Moon*, an illustrated poem about laying the foundations of a life in tune with nature: 'May the morning sun warm you, the evening breeze cool you, and at noon may you rest in the shade.' Simple things we shouldn't take for granted – much like good health.

Vida's palate expands (slightly) to encompass chickpeas, pasta with Marmite, and celery. Gabriel is weaned on sweet potato and scrambled egg, and he evolves into a fruit bat of a child. His eyes light up at his first taste of orange. He eats hungrily, trustingly, without Vida's tinge of suspicion about food, which is hardly surprising, given my cunning attempts to sneak medicine into what she eats and drinks. They both have banana porridge for breakfast, and we continue to sprinkle the chelation med over Vida's to remove at least some of the iron which will now be building up in her system.

In the spring, when Gabriel is a few months old, and just after Vida turns two, she has her much-anticipated steroid trial, which has been held up by Covid. We hope it works, without expecting it to, and it doesn't. These are the hardest four weeks we have had since she was a baby. She becomes a hungrier, more bullish version of herself, and hardly sleeps. As these drugs will weaken her immune system, we isolate and are again presented with the singular challenge of shielding a child who is, quite literally, a toddler on steroids. Freddie and I are disturbed by the experience; by this point, we have known Vida mostly well and stable with regular blood transfusions. But during the trial, her transfusions are paused and she is monitored to see if the steroids kickstart her bone marrow. Vida's reticulocytes stay the same – practically zero – and her haemoglobin dwindles to a worrying low. With this she looks grey; she cries, gets inexplicably angry. I have never been so pleased to see a cannula and a bag of blood as when the hospital makes the call to transfuse her. The trial is called a failure. At least now we know.

In the autumn she starts at a local nursery called Chelwood. It's a special place: children roam freely between classes and about the playground, which is set up differently each day with foam and sand, chalk and water play, tyre swings and elevated tunnels, vats of conkers in autumn, curling courgette flowers in summer and the most giant sunflowers I've ever seen. Music thuds quietly through an outdoor speaker. There is a perennial feeling of joy here and, frankly, I'd like to stay and play too. Chelwood is not really a 'childcare solution' – Vida stays for just under three hours every morning at first – but we feel instinctively that it will be a good place for her, and for Gabriel later.

Over time, she starts to make friends. Her teachers know that she has a bone-marrow transplant on the horizon and they laminate photographs of hospital settings, which they tack to the wall in a corner of the classroom. They leave a doctor's kit and some dolls nearby. It is in this corner that Vida strikes up a friendship with one girl in particular, a girl who also has a condition that requires regular hospital visits. They listen to each other's heartbeats, take temperatures, administer medicines and cannulas, offer each other reassurance. I am bowled over by the power of play, and the importance of shared experience, even at three years old.

∽

Vida had her bone-marrow transplant at St Mary's hospital when she had just turned four, on 8 March 2023. That it was International Women's Day was a fluke, but it felt like a good omen. A transplant marks a new chapter for the patient, a new lease of life in the truest sense, and its date becomes another birthday. And not only one for Vida: 8 March is also the day that two-year-old Gabriel makes his donation. For twenty-four hours, all four of us will be in hospital.

How to write about our son's part in it all? We have avoided allusions to 'saviour' status, but he is, for us, the unknowing hero. We have gone only as far as to tell Vida that Gabes is 'sharing some of his blood' with her. She is concerned about him 'going to sleep', having his blood removed; we tell her that he has lots of it, that he won't remember, that he will be OK. We say this to remind ourselves, too. Amid my pragmatism, I must also remember the cost of this to Gabriel. Older siblings would have had to have counselling before becoming a donor. Until now, Freddie and I have minimised the significance of what he will have to endure – the many blood tests, the general anaesthetic, the soreness in his lower back where the bone marrow will be taken, and the consequent anaemia which will require months of iron supplementation. It was doubtless more acceptable to us because we have lived with Vida having these same procedures and symptoms time and again. Still, we are signing up our baby for the possibility of pain and distress. This doesn't sit comfortably.

There are systems in place to protect Gabriel in all of this, however. He has his own consultant to assess his fitness to donate and to represent his interests. Freddie and I also have several rounds of counselling with Becky, the clinical psychologist at St Mary's; what, she asks, are the benefits to Gabriel of the procedure? Our response is stark: to have a sister who is in the best possible health for the longest possible time. Their fiery squabbles notwithstanding, we see the bond between our kids. The way that, if Vida is given a snack or a toy, she'll always ask if there's one for 'Bao' (unable to say 'Gabriel', this is what she calls him for his first two years, a nickname Freddie and I embrace too, as he does have something of a delicious steamed bun about him). The way that, when we pick him up from his childminder, the first thing Gabriel asks is always, 'Where's Vida?' The way that, when we play music in the car, he watches and copies her moves and chants with a gleeful grin. We believe Gabriel would choose to do this for Vida if he could, and that one day he will be proud to know he changed the course of her life, of our family life. Separating the children for a long period will be hard, but we feel clear about the pay-off – for Gabriel as well as for Vida.

Two weeks before the transplant, Vida moves into her hospital cubicle for a fortnight of IV medications and Gabriel is relocated to Louise's house in West Hampstead. We have no idea how long Vida will be living here; we've psyched ourselves up for three months, hoping for less but accepting the very real possibility that it could be more. I have taken an indefinite period of parental leave from work. The plan is for Freddie and me to take it in turns to spend the night with her (while the other sleeps with Gabriel at Louise's). Every morning, whoever has slept in West Hampstead returns with laundered bed sheets, a Tupperware of leftovers, and an array of snacks for Vida, because experience tells us she is likely to refuse hospital food.

Gabriel spends his days with one of his grannies or a part-time nanny we have found for extra help. He adapts well to the routine, enjoying visits to the library, a ball pit in a local church, and Camden's many playgrounds. Being just twenty minutes from the hospital makes it possible for Freddie and me both to spend time with each of our children every day – as transplant set-ups go for a family of four, they don't come much better than this, although I'm conscious of how strange and difficult it must be for Gabriel, in less obvious ways than for Vida. Siblings in these situations are sometimes referred to as the 'shadow patients', their relative health in some ways putting them at a disadvantage. Throughout the BMT, we are conscious of this and try to compensate for it, but there's also no getting round the toll that Vida's procedure will take on her brother.

At the hospital, we are pleasantly surprised by Vida's cubicle. It is accessed via an 'anteroom' from the corridor, a little space in which hands are washed and sanitised and full, fresh PPE is put on by whoever comes in. It has two beds, two chairs, a desk, a shelving unit and a fridge, with plenty of floor space left over. As soon as we're in, we put up a noticeboard on the desk and put up photos from home – one of Gabriel and Vida together on the beach in Norfolk last summer, another of a sleepy-looking Ernie, and a picture of us as a family outside our house, the last one taken before the big move into hospital – Gabriel's is still baby hair, soft and white-blonde, Vida has a straight chestnut bob, which I know she will lose soon.

We try to keep Vida active in hospital from the off, knowing that she is likely to feel less like moving as time wears on, and that inactivity can lead to muscle wastage. Freddie has bought her a wobble board and we try to use a playmat as much as possible, tipping out tubs of Playmobil or magnetic building tiles to work and rework into different structures. On the rare occasion that Vida isn't attached to a line, I try to get her to dance (she loves Katy Perry) and discover a My Little Pony yoga class on YouTube.

On the same day that she is admitted, Vida has a nasogastric (NG) tube and her Hickman line fitted. The Hickman is a tube placed in a vein in her chest, which then divides into three lines or 'lumens' which dangle from her tiny torso. Before it is fitted, we are daunted by how it will make her, and us, feel to see it, such a tangible symbol of her situation. But we quickly become strangely fond of her 'wigglies', as she calls it, offering easy, long-term access to her veins. Through the Hickman, she receives the many medicines she needs, and has blood drawn for daily testing. Vida is troubled less by the drama of this new, foreign thing emerging from her body than by the dressing over it, which needs to be changed weekly. It as an ordeal for her, the stripping away of adhesive painful, but it is vital that we keep it squeaky clean to avoid infection – and we will rely on the Hickman for everything in the upcoming acute phase: chemotherapy, antibodies, transfusions of red blood cells and platelets, immunosuppressants and prophylactic meds, and Gabriel's stem cells.

True to the idea of having a second birthday, transplant day is named 'Day 0'. Everything which came before is a minus number, and each day after is a plus: Day +1, +2, and so forth. I like the positivity of this trajectory – that we are heading upwards in numbers – although I do not want to lose sight of what came before. While there will of course be a before and an after, a reason to refer to 'pre-' and 'post-transplant', neither Freddie nor myself believe in 'the other side' to all this. When Vida was newly diagnosed, my hope had been that a bone-marrow transplant would provide a gateway to moving on; now I look at things a little differently. While I know life won't always be this extraordinary exertion, our experience with Diamond-Blackfan has by now been folded into who we are. I no longer see Vida's transplant as setting us back on course for a life that her diagnosis rerouted. It is, quite simply, the thing we are doing to give her the best life that modern medicine can. There was the life I imagined and the life that is. I'm interested in the latter.

In the months leading up to this, I have been mostly upbeat, at peace with the decision to go ahead and spurred on by a sense of purpose. Today, however, six days before the transplant, I have my first and only real wobble: Vida is starting her 'conditioning' treatment: a cocktail of meds, including chemotherapy, which will destroy her bone-marrow cells in preparation for Gabriel's. Once she has received her first dose of chemo, there is no going back (several months back, I signed a contract confirming that I understood this). Two nurses enter our cubicle: one is our designated carer for the day; the other is specially trained in administering chemo and wears, in addition to PPE, a thick apron and gloves as she handles a red bag of liquid with toxicity warnings written across it. Suddenly I see my responsibility in sharp relief. Who are Freddie and I to decide whether our child should have this treatment? We're only her parents! It feels like only yesterday that *we* were children.

We FaceTime Gabriel and Louise before the chemo begins. It is lunchtime and she is feeding him poached chicken and vegetables, which he's eating voraciously. Our mums have pre-emptively taken it upon themselves to feed Gabes up with iron-boosting foods before his bone-marrow donation: stocks made from boiled meat bones, steak from the butcher, my mum has even made him liver cupcakes. 'Hi Vida!' he cries, showing her a roaring dragon toy Louise found him at the charity shop. I know how important these calls are, keeping the communication lines open between our kids, but they are bittersweet and reinforce our unnatural separation. Louise is jolly, recounting to Vida what she and Gabriel did that morning, and how she is looking forward to doing all those same things with her when she comes home. She doesn't let on how hard this must be for her. If Gabriel is the shadow patient, the grandparents are the shadow carers, I think, rallying to care for Gabes and stay positive for us all, their own fears and exhaustion marginalised in the collective effort. Everyone's breath is held, whale-like, for as long as this takes.

After the call, I take a moment in the anteroom, lean on the basin, let out a sob. I dab at my eyes with coarse dispenser paper, only to realise I am crying without tears. I always think there is relief in a decision made, and I reason that once the first dose is in, my panic will ease, as it often does. But it feels so inappropriate, self-indulgent even, to apply such flippant rationale: this is my daughter's life. There is an alternative: a lifetime of transfusions and iron chelation. But I've done my reading. I've spoken to other families. I know why we're doing this. I look through the small window into the cubicle, at my girl with her bobbed hair and cheeks still toddler-plump – features that this procedure will see off, for now – and steel myself. Is that a cliché? Maybe. I've had four years to build up to this, though, and now is the moment to jump.

The six days of conditioning are less dramatic than I had expected. The chemo goes in, her appetite fades gradually, and for now her hair stays rooted to her head. On Day −4, it is actually not a chemo drug but an antibody derived from rabbits known as ATG that makes her the most unwell she's been, spiking a high fever. The night doctor and nurses stabilise her quickly with paracetamol and morphine and, by morning, she is weak but cheery when I give her a present. Our friend Boo has brought her a bag full of little things wrapped in brown paper – books, stickers, a paperweight with a four-leaf clover inside it. Vida has always been picky enough about food that it isn't a very good gauge of whether she feels well or not. Presents, however, she is seldom ambivalent about. If she perks up at a present, I'm not overly worried.

On Day 0, Freddie wakes up with Vida in hospital. I get up with Gabriel in West Hampstead, dressing him but skipping breakfast – he has been nil by mouth since the night before in anticipation of his big moment. It is finally here, and it feels surreal because these are motions that I have only gone through with Vida before now. We arrive for 7 a.m.; Gabes moans at me for snacks. We are both in tracksuits. I pull Gabes's Mickey Mouse sweatshirt over his luminous head of hair and swap it for a hospital gown strewn with teddy-bear pictures. Shirlei, the play therapist, who we have come to know well in the lead-up to transplant, brings him some felt-tips and a *Toy Story* line drawing to colour in. A softly spoken anaesthetist comes to remind me of all the risks of what we are about to do. I have heard all this many times before, but it is still unnerving.

Neither of my kids take things lying down (quite literally) and both can be vocal in their protests. But Gabriel's objections manifest differently from his sister's. Where Vida's tears in hospital tend to be of fear, knowing from experience what might be about to happen; Gabriel's are hot and angry, incensed that anyone might try to restrain him while brandishing a stethoscope or, worse, a needle. And while experience sees Vida bounce back fast from the likes of a blood test, Gabes's mood stays bruised by the interventions of a doctor or nurse. He tells me that he didn't like 'dat red night' (the sats monitor), or 'dat sharp fing'. He has the stubbornness of a mule and the memory of an elephant; this is apt because it is during this period that he becomes entranced by 'Colonel Hathi's March' from *The Jungle Book*. If I can't get him to walk in the direction I want – up the hallway, through the park, down a hospital corridor – I break into 'Hup, two, three, four' and we drill our way there.

When the moment comes to place the mask over his face and watch him drop off, I falter. My sweet, sparky, wilful boy. When in the past I have watched Vida go through the same, my sadness has been about our lack of choice in the matter – the injustice of her condition. But in Gabriel's case, we are choosing this, opting in. Like the first dose of chemo, my responsibility is dizzyingly apparent. Freddie and I have an agency in all of this for which we feel criminally underqualified. Four years ago, I couldn't have told you what a stem cell was.

Gabriel's stem-cell donation is abundant, Josu tells us afterwards (Josu had arranged his schedule so that he could personally retrieve the marrow and be present for Vida's transplant). After the procedure, Gabes is given a cubicle next door to Vida's on Grand Union ward. His big eyes are hooded in sleep, but he is otherwise upbeat, enthused by the Marmite cheese biscuits my mum has dropped off for him at reception. He plays with a large plastic truck full of glow-in-the-dark dinosaur figurines given to him by a friend. A tag on it reads 'For the bravest boy'. Meanwhile, his stem cells are en route to Hammersmith Hospital, where they will be processed before being returned late afternoon, ready to enter their new home, Vida.

A bone-marrow transplant is not an operation but a process. The actual transplant itself, the moment when the donor's cells enter the recipient's body over the period of a couple of hours, is a tiny proportion of the many months or even years it can take for the process to be finished. There's also a hint of anticlimax to it for a family so familiar with blood transfusions; indeed, for Vida, the moment her bone-marrow transplant happens is indistinguishable from a transfusion. It is a bag of deep-red liquid – a richer, more potent elixir than the blood she has always been transfused with, but she doesn't know that – which is hooked up to her Hickman line. And that's it.

It happens at about 6 p.m. It is bathtime at home, just one of many daily examples of how time is reframed in hospital. We have a family photo of it beginning: I am grinning, euphoric. I remember the feeling in my chest, full like the helium balloons behind Vida's bed, one of them a 'V', the other a 'G'. Next to me is Josu, his eyes betraying the smile under his mask. Flanking the other side of the bed are a sleepy Gabriel in his robe, and Freddie, who is evidently overwhelmed. In the middle is Vida. She smiles widely on her bed with its pink unicorn covers; it is unusual for her to pose so willingly. Perhaps it was the sheer pleasure of having her family restored around her. Or maybe on some level she knew what this moment could mean for the rest of her life.

—

Doctors keep reminding us that the side effects of chemotherapy are cumulative, gradual, and as time passes, we see this for ourselves in the dwindling appeal of marshmallows and Percy Pigs. There are days when Vida takes herself to bed for naps (unheard of, normally) – but never to her own patient bed, with its remote control, flip-down sides and lockable wheels. By day, Freddie and I make the metal fold-out one intended for parents into a daybed, covering it with a throw to protect it from drink spills and paint sticks. Vida calls it 'the little bed', or even 'my bed', and insists on sleeping in it, day and night, for the first few weeks until the nurse in charge insists otherwise. It's considerably less comfortable than the patient bed, but that's irrelevant. She doesn't see herself as a patient.

We were warned of mucositis, the painful inflammation of the digestive tract that happens after chemo. This starts a few days afterwards with mouth ulcers and lip sores, which then progress down through her system. Four times a day we have to clean her mouth with Corsodyl to relieve it; four times a day she protests. Around this time, she is put onto supplementary nutrition in two forms: a foul-smelling milk that is shot from a suspended bag into her NG tube at regular intervals, and TPN (total parenteral nutrition), which she receives intravenously. Together, they keep her weight on, and her digestive system working, through a period when food and even drink are anathema to her.

Every day since chemo started, I have gently tested the roots of Vida's hair to see if it is loosening from her scalp.

On Day +7, a few hairs shred into my fingers. The following morning, I notice that her pillowcase has more of her maroon strands across it. I tug gently at it during the day, mesmerised by the ease with which it falls. Sometimes she doesn't notice, at others it irritates her. I just want it out now, because once it's gone, all we will have to do is wait for it to return: the hair loss, the big outward show of Vida's transplant, will be in the past. On Day +9, after more pillow hair, Freddie suggests to Vida that he shaves her head with his beard trimmer. I am surprised when she agrees so readily. She sits on the daybed in a unicorn dress with a tulle skirt. While her dad mows her hair off, she sits calmly, quizzically looking at the handfuls that fall into her lap. Afterwards, we pass her a hand mirror. She looks into it, observes her head from different angles. She smiles, purses her lips, lets out a giggle. What a kid.

Now that she has received Gabriel's cells, it's a waiting game. While her immune system is non-existent, she stays isolated in the hospital cubicle and is monitored. Every day for the next few weeks, we will track the numbers. We need her neutrophils – the most numerous of white blood cells in the human body, and that help it fight infections – to be over 0.5 for three days running for her to be termed 'engrafted'. Every morning, I request a printout of her 6 a.m. bloods and wait nervously for this fortune-telling sheet to arrive with a nurse.

On Day +13, we have our third day above 0.5. This is within the timeframe they expected, and it is our first indication that things are heading in the right direction. It is an epic game of snakes and ladders, and today we have climbed some vital rungs.

It is strange to have been so preoccupied with red blood cells and haemoglobin for four years, and suddenly to speak so little of them. Right now, talk is all of neutrophils and lymphocytes or platelets.

Before her transplant, I had become used to following Vida's blood counts and infection markers, and it became a compulsion. This has only intensified with the BMT. I grow addicted to the sense of progress that following the numbers gives me. I have so little control over any of this, yet each climbing cell count feels like a major achievement. I've not had such a feeling of forward motion about Vida's health before. Transfusion life was a three-week-long carousel before she needed blood again, but if her counts continue along this trajectory, she may never need another transfusion.

Gabriel was sent home the morning after his donation. A blood test showed he was anaemic, which we'd expected, as around his eyes, lips and ears we can see that same pallor we've come to recognise in Vida. In the following weeks, we feed him a cherry-flavoured iron supplement three times a day, and his haemoglobin becomes normal again within a couple of months.

I feel immense pride in my children's bodies. Not many parents know what their children's reticulocyte counts are, much less need to celebrate them. Slanted motherhood this might be, but it certainly has some beautiful angles.

Even in the midst of Hickman lines and nasogastric tubes, bedpans and beeping, when sleep is scarce and we worry about how the next few months will go, there are moments when

I feel privileged to be having this experience with my children. We see each other in ways that most families never will; separated we may be, but bonded too. Like when Vida tells people that Gabriel shared his blood with her. Or the family FaceTime calls between the hospital room and Gabriel's bathtime, when they show each other new toys and bubbles, books read and pictures drawn, and when he makes her giggle with what she has come to understand as him being a toddler. These calls can be hard, too, of course; the few occasions when Vida's chemotherapy-induced nausea makes her too subdued to talk, or when she says under her breath, 'But I want to be at Louise's house,' and, 'Are we going to live here forever?' There's the time when Gabriel first sees her with an NG tube and cries. There's the feeling, for Freddie and me, that we are always somewhere we should be but can't be, divided as we and our children are between two places.

There are days during Vida's inpatient stay when I am amazed by things I see incidentally. St Mary's hospital is situated beside Paddington Basin and our room on Grand Union ward overlooks the canal for which it is named. By day, the area bustles with activity. Tourists amble down to Little Venice. Commuters make their way to work, sipping flat whites with their eyes glued to phone screens. The hospital is opposite the Marks & Spencer offices, and we gradually deduce their working patterns: Tuesdays and Thursdays seem to be office days, when through glass walls we see them gathered around conference tables. By night, it's a ghost town, surprisingly so given our central location. It's just us and a handful of barges below. I have always loved names – naming dogs, babies, the names of places, houses, boats. Barges are no exception, and it is during the early days of Vida's admission, when she has high doses of chemotherapy every day, that one name in particular jumps out at me. SANGUINE, it reads. Sanguine, meaning 'blood red' in old English. Sanguine, meaning, according to the *Oxford English Dictionary*, 'optimistic or positive, especially in an apparently bad or difficult situation'. I have spent these last years trying not to look for signs, but I can't say I'm not heartened by this. It is a wave of reassurance from somewhere. I have seen for myself that blood is power, in deed and now in word.

Having made such a strong relationship with St Thomas' Hospital, we had been apprehensive about the move to St Mary's. We needn't have been. Not only are they the experts in this procedure, but we quickly grow to know and love the staff. I am humbled by the nurses on Grand Union, all of whom have chosen to work in this particularly intense area of medicine. Bone-marrow transplants involve not only making children more unwell before they can get better, but inevitably include navigating anxious, often confused, and angry parents. The staff handle us nimbly and with empathy, but they always make sure they address Vida too; they get down to her level and include all four years of her in the process.

When someone enters the cubicle with a cardboard dish of syringes containing multicoloured suspensions, or a plastic tray of dressings or blood vials, Vida panics and cries, but is – after the event – often placated with play, like stringing plastic bead necklaces together, or by showing them a new toy. She is entering a phase of girlhood, one that I remember for myself, when some young women are the objects of fascination. For

Vida, it's nurses Ristell and Habiba in particular who she asks for by name. But we grow to appreciate things about all the nurses – each with their different strengths, boundaries and tenderness. We feel we come to know many of them well; we learn about their families or where they live, how they ended up working on a bone-marrow transplant ward. Perversely, though, we know only half of their faces. We get to know hairlines or headscarves, brows and eyes, jewellery and shoes, but from nose to jaw, these women are a mystery to us. On the occasions that I leave the cubicle and see them on reception without their masks, I am alarmed by the unexpected contours of nostrils, lips, chins. Just one of the little weirdnesses of the life we are living.

Suddenly, we are allowed to go home. It shouldn't really feel sudden – it is Day +24 and we have lived in this cubicle for five and a half weeks. It is also the first day of April, and so for a moment we wonder if it is all a joke. But they tell us that Vida's progress is good and stable enough for her to become an outpatient. We will need to come back to St Mary's two days a week for the time being.

Clearing out the cubicle is like moving house. We have so much stuff: obvious things like bedding, and then *everything else*. Pen lids and plastic gemstones, bags of crisps, painkillers and dumbbells, crates of Playmobil and a Velcro dartboard, lots of books, and I can't even tell you how many stickers.

We have been told to prepare for a year out of mainstream life and that Vida is likely to be on immunosuppressant medication for many months, which comes hand in hand with lots of other prophylactic drugs. I am given a lesson in measuring up the medications. So far, this has all been done for us, first in the form of intravenous meds, and then, when it was time to try giving them to her orally, the nurses supplied us with loaded syringes. For all the stresses of the last six weeks, we have had an enormous amount of support from the team here. As predicted, Vida has not got to the point where she can take all nine meds in her mouth multiple times a day, and is heading home with an NG tube. It's far from ideal. So I am being schooled not just in measuring up, but in administering meds down the tube. This involves drawing back some stomach fluid through the NG with a large syringe and then testing the pH: if it is below 5.5, the tube is definitely in place in her stomach and the meds can be given. Once all of them have gone in (not always easy, she hates the sensation), we flush the last one through with sterile water.

When the car is loaded up, the time comes for Vida to leave Grand Union. It is inevitable that we will be back over the coming months, but we know that an era has come to an end. The nurses are lined up waiting for her to ring the bell, which signals that the first inpatient stage of treatment is done. (Further down the line, when it is all over, she will ring another bell of greater significance.) Everyone cheers. She is taken behind the reception desk and cuddled, even allowed into the doctors' office, where a few cherished kids' artworks for the team are tacked up. Vida already has one there. She has won some hearts in this place.

Outside, Vida is all appreciation. 'I love my car,' she says as we strap her in. 'Can I smell the air?' she asks, as we pull away from the hospital. We open the window a crack: spring air plus the scent of Edgware Road. Freddie swings down to Marble Arch, where the daffodils are out – 'Daffodils!' she cries. 'They're like trumpets!' And they are, I think, brightly proclaiming her release. By the time we reach the bottom of Park Lane, she is asleep, and stays that way until we get home.

Louise brings Gabriel back within the hour. He runs into the hallway and Vida opens the living-room door. They stand and look at each other, four and two years old, grinning. They don't quite know what to do.

'It's nice to see you, Vida.'

'It's so nice to see you too!'

They start to play, and at this sight, a part of me that had broken is welded back together.

During the summer of 2023 we celebrate our relative freedom – our own beds! a kitchen! glasses of wine! – but are tethered to hospital and live in strict isolation. Freddie is able to go to work, as his team is small, but the kids and I must avoid infections and stay at home. The hospital have said that Gabriel should continue to have a life outside of the house, but we reason that sending him to nursery now would be madness. We really don't need him bringing bugs home, so we find a part-time nanny to take him out, mostly to parks, on Vida's hospital days.

Everyone knows that small children are germ magnets and put everything in their mouths. Mine are no exception. For all our efforts at keeping surfaces clean, hands washed and exposure to other people limited, there remain unknown quantities. We become acutely aware of all the risks we cannot see. Vida's new immune system is very immature and will struggle to fight viruses for a long time. The Hickman line also presents an infection risk. We are instructed to bring her to hospital for IV antibiotics if ever she has a temperature over 38°C, to ward off the risk of a septic line infection. Luckily, the summer weather and our isolation conspire to keep Vida pretty well in our first few months at home, and our regular hospital visits are reserved for monitoring and planned meds.

During the long commutes to and from Paddington, I window-shop other people's lives. Through Camberwell, Elephant and Castle, Victoria, I ogle their quotidian freedoms: to enter Tube stations, cafés, office buildings; to take their children to school, to museums, to socialise; to wear something other than a tracksuit and Crocs.

I have gone from feeling like a citizen of the world to a citizen of my house. Summer can be a cruel season for families dealing with disabilities, as I know from the year Vida was diagnosed. I stay on Instagram, determined to keep my toe dipped in the outside world, but it is often unhelpful, as the lives I see there contrast so drastically to our own. As the months warm up, my friends and acquaintances start going on holiday. I don't envy their destinations because I know we have travel in our future. In this I can be single-minded – what we are doing now is a passport to all of that. What I find harder is the seeming ease with which I see people travel with their young children. Babies on planes, toddlers kicking their feet on lapping shorelines, family meals of local foods... a bit of me mourns the experiences we have lost to the pandemic and now to transplant. It is for Vida and Gabriel, not myself, that I feel sad, though. And I know I must keep my eyes on the prize.

I think about privilege a lot. There is a dearth of financial and pastoral support for parents of children who have chronic conditions, most of all when treatment affects a parent's ability to work. I have had to take an indefinite period of unpaid leave for Vida's transplant and money is tight, but I also know how fortunate we are. We live in London and have easy access to the specialist hospital; we have a house with a garden, so even though Vida can't go to parks, she can at least be outside; we are tapping into savings to fund some part-time childcare help, because the kids' needs are so very different right now. And frankly, I don't know how I'd manage them both on my own every day, such are the demands of Vida's medicine and personal hygiene regime, and Gabriel's energetic toddlerdom.

I also see health privilege now. A privilege Vida has never had and which, by proxy, we no longer have either. What must it be like to move so freely through the world as a parent? I yearn for the day that I take my children to a swimming pool or a party. Even to give them a bath together, which the Hickman line, for now, does not permit; every night, Vida has a quick shower to avoid wetting her dressing while Gabriel splashes luxuriously in the tub. This is health privilege starkly in action, as is Gabriel's freedom to eat raspberries, nuts, raw dairy, cured meat, and even to drink tap water (Vida can only drink water that has been boiled and then cooled). Every aspect of her day is monitored, curated, limited somehow. My children have in so many ways had the same upbringing, yet for all of Gabriel's brushes with the hospital, there is so much about Vida's experience of the world that he will never know.

Transfusion life has become a thing of the past, at least. Vida last had a bag of red cells just a couple of days before she was discharged and, as the weeks roll on, this feels nothing short of a miracle. Before transplant, she would have gone into sharp decline after four weeks without blood; now her haemoglobin is stable and her reticulocytes not just present, but high in number. Stability brings waves of both euphoria and grief for me. Mostly the former – I am happy and encouraged by the way things are going – but on occasion I will fall upon a photo of a younger Vida evidently in need of a transfusion. I remember how she had kicked and screamed at cannulation, and how I had learnt to hold it together, and I feel a kind of delayed distress about it all. Distance casts a different shade on things.

The to-ing and fro-ing to hospital is tiring, but the closest thing that Vida or I have to a social event. She loves seeing the nurses, showing them her outfits, her toys, and I am relieved to have direct contact with people who are knowledgeable about all of this. Our two days a week at St Mary's give us a framework. Are we institutionalised? Yes, probably; going to hospital now feels in some ways like going to the office did post-Covid. I've gone from hybrid working to hybrid caring.

Isolation at home, empty of routine except for mealtimes and Gabriel's nap, makes me think of the slime that Vida learnt to make with the play specialist on Grand Union. Freddie went back to work in April and while I have part-time support from nannies and grannies, a lot of the care falls to me. Most of the time, I feel less like their mother than a referee. Vida might be vulnerable, but in tussles over toys she gives as good as she's got.

So does Gabriel, who may still be shorter than his sister but is now heavier. The all-time low comes in May when he pulls out her NG tube. This feels nothing short of a disaster – we rely on the tube for almost all her meds. It is the evening and Freddie is at a work event. I measure up the syringes and implore Vida to try taking them orally while Gabriel climbs on me, *miaows*, and claws at my boobs. He's been weaned for a year but I resort to letting him pretend to breastfeed so I can focus on Vida taking her life-saving medicine. I know I will laugh about it later, but in that moment it feels spectacularly bleak.

The NG is replaced only the once, but we develop new strategies for getting Vida to take stuff just in case. Over many months, she starts to take her immunosuppressants with dwindling resistance, blackmailed by promises to stay up later than Gabes, eat sprinkles, get presents, including a life-size Barbie head whose hair can be styled (we call her Terry, short for Terrifying). We give Vida some of the other medicines in a bottle of milk once she is half asleep. There is nothing like the sound of a sleeping child drinking milk – is there anything cosier than the nose breaths, the soft swallows? To hear it makes me feel swaddled myself. I am reminded in these moments of how reciprocal nurturing a child can be. In some ways, parenting is not as one-sided as we are led to think.

For five years, life has ticked to the rhythms of love and science. Our friend Boo remarked early on in Vida's big admission that it was these two things which would get us through, and it's a mantra I've kept in mind. Love and science, love and science, love and science.

—

The challenges of Vida's treatment evolved over time, but the intensity didn't. In the autumn of the transplant year, I went back to work after eight months off and it gave me relief and pressure in equal measure. How lovely for my brain to escape into food, but how hideous the juggle. Vida's immune system became stronger, and she started to be given little freedoms – play dates with well children, a pizza in an empty restaurant, and eventually, she started school – but freedom can have a sting in its tail. School means bugs, bugs mean temperatures and, as she had a Hickman line until the following March, temperatures mean hospital admissions. Whenever she had a fever, we moved into St Mary's at a moment's notice for days-long courses of antibiotics; I'd do video calls for work from the ward with its cacophony of alarms while Vida – who usually felt well – created an obstacle course on the adjustable bed beside me. This happened about every week for a couple of months.

Our story arc is, so far, a satisfying one. A child with a serious diagnosis for whom invasive treatment has proved successful. Getting here has been hard work, but it also feels like the work has only just begun. Since the Hickman line was removed and Vida's immunosuppressant medication has stopped, her life has properly opened up. After a very stop-and-start introduction to school, she attended for the entire summer term and loved it. Now for blending letters into words! Making friends! Healthy eating! I love the ordinariness of it all. This kind of hard work – the, dare I say it, 'normal' stuff – is what we've dreamt of for so long.

We're told that stories have a beginning, a middle and an end, but now that Vida has had her transplant, I feel done with endings. I am in the fortunate position of my daughter having come through treatment successfully, but I also think that in the past I have, perhaps, been too attached to fixed outcomes – such as what having children would be like. While my heart ached for things to be different, for Vida not to need all these interventions, I nonetheless have two happy children. I've met people I'd otherwise never have, and forged friendships on an understanding that's almost as rare as DBA itself. I have been humbled and astounded by the National Health Service and its people – who don't just bring science, but love, to the nth degree. I have been reminded time and again of what community looks like, from the indefatigable loyalty of our parents to the kindness of people we hardly know. There has been joy in all of this middle bit. Perhaps our story will now be an eternal middle, a life where we can live in the moment. Love and science have afforded us that.

In the early years I was devastated by how different parenthood was playing out from what I'd imagined. But five years in, I don't want another version of life with Vida and Gabriel. I don't need them to be early talkers or prodigious readers, keen swimmers or aspiring astronauts, teachers, vets. I just want them to be. For them to be here, for them to be well. For us to keep being in the middle.

September 2024

Outside the women's loo in paediatric haematology is a bell. It's an old-fashioned school one, with a wide mouth and a rope hanging from its clapper. Next to it there is a plaque, which bears these words:

> Ring this bell
> three times well
> its toll to clearly say
> my treatment's done
> this course is run
> and I am on my way!

I never allowed myself to think about the bell too much, especially in the early years, knowing how many obstacles stood between Vida and a life without transfusions. Sometimes, though, we'd see other children ring it, and I'd well up at the thought of Vida standing beneath it one day while someone read out the poem.

In the end, that someone was me. It was June of this year, 2024. Watching the video back, I read with a voice that becomes steadily louder, a crescendo to compete with Vida's bellows of, 'CAN I RING IT NOW? CAN I RING IT?' Standing on a table, underneath the bell, she wears her school uniform, with her hair, now not-quite-bob length, in a comical topknot to keep a growing forelock out of her eyes. By her side: her bone-marrow angel, Gabriel. He wasn't going to miss out on the chance to give the bell a ring either. They were ready to declare, together, their freedom from the tyranny of immunosuppressants. On paediatric wards, bells do not toll for the dead – they proclaim the living.

It was of course a happy day, but a strange one too. It meant that we would be seeing less of our medical team – down from twice a week to once a month at first, then every quarter, then twice a year and, eventually, just annually. We would miss them. The truth is that Vida loves going to hospital. And having watched the two of us pack up to go there so many times, Gabriel has become fascinated by it too, often looking for reasons why he himself might need to go. Hospital, in his mind, makes you special – a place of unbridled screen time, bottomless snacks and cool stickers.

In the lead-up to ringing the bell, I had been focused on it being The End. But it's really a beginning: *I am on my way*. Not least because with Vida's health – or really, with anyone's – there are no hard endings. The definitive 'fix' I once craved for her doesn't exist, nor does it for anyone. Vida will need more monitoring during her life than the 'average' person (whatever that means), but while any of us have life, our health hangs over us like a question mark.

Would I change what has happened? Now I can't fathom a life in which it hadn't. Certainly, I don't dream wistfully of a version without Diamond-Blackfan anaemia. It is what it is and so much more. I suppose I have developed respect for the genetic code that has moulded my family so uniquely. Without it, I wouldn't have the two kids I do.

The final months of Vida's transplant had been some of the hardest, when the snakes-and-ladders analogy felt more apt than ever. She was weaned off one of her immunosuppressants and allowed to start school in January, quickly making friends and forming a close bond with her class teacher. But she was still on one potent drug, and she still had a Hickman line. Surrounded by hundreds of other children, Vida quickly caught every bug going and had to be readmitted to hospital with a temperature almost every week, staying for several days at a time so she could be treated for sepsis preventatively. It was disruptive for everyone, and especially hard on Gabriel.

While Vida would quickly feel better and spend forty-eight hours watching Disney and filling sticker books with me, our three-year-old boy would lose his mum and sister without warning and, to him, inexplicably. There was one particularly long and bad admission when he was himself sick at home – sicker than Vida in hospital. We called our nanny so we could speak to him and he looked forlorn, with sunken eyes and a runny nose. 'I miss my family,' he said under his breath.

Gabriel had adapted to the military drill of transplant life well at the beginning, when he had only just turned two. But once we were sent home, the procedure became more chaotic and harder to plan, and this corresponded with his own rapidly developing needs. I could see that a routine would help him to feel safe, but bone-marrow transplant demands that routines are abandoned; if Vida showed the slightest sign of a fever, A & E it was. That, inevitably, has taken a toll on a chunk of Gabriel's earliest years. We are making space for his recovery, too.

Water has been the defining element of this past spring and summer at our house. Since Vida's Hickman line was removed in March, bathtimes, swimming trips and the paddling pool have been restored to daily life. The children's ability to submerge themselves together is progress in its realest form, bodies of water our totems of change. The first times they did these things together again were poignant, but quickly normalised, the flooding of the bathroom floor – from a water fight that got out of hand, say, or a tussle over a flannel – shaking me out of grateful reflection to mop up.

Without the Hickman, Vida can now also get herself dressed, and she revels in planning her outfits for the days ahead, laying out leggings and T-shirts with clashing prints, careful never to forget a rainbow of accessories. She has a new love of food and has discovered halloumi, pasta with any kind of pulse, and a host of retro puddings. At school she is known for her confidence, for having a big voice and a big heart, and for often breaking into song in the playground.

Gabriel, meanwhile, is a man of passions, which include prehistoric creatures, amphibians and combine harvesters. 'Mummy, I'm looking for some inspiration,' he told me the other day, something he never actually seems short of, but I can tell he is ready for his world to open up. He has been hot-headed in the last few months, perhaps on some level knowing it is now safe to act out some of his distress. We have moved him to the nursery at Vida's school, so that they share a routine, scooting round the corner to the school gates together each morning while I, their concierge, lug bags and coats behind them.

And what of Freddie and me? We squirrelled away a bottle of champagne several years ago, saving it to toast the bell ringing, and we still haven't popped its cork, drunk its bubbles. Why not? There are boring, practical reasons, of course: the big day happened on the Wednesday of a busy week, Freddie had a sore throat, yada yada yada. But given we've had three months in which to celebrate since, I know there's another reason. Daily life is celebration enough, its ordinariness the greatest luxury. After the brief thrill of ringing the bell, Vida was onto the next thing, and so are we. We are swimming with the current, the pulse of our lifeblood propelling us forward into the beautiful unknown ahead.

Acknowledgements

I started writing this book a year into motherhood, twelve months in which life as I knew it erupted into something unrecognisable. It was during that time – a time when I thought I might never write another word – that I met with Ariella Feiner at United Agents. What luck, for me. She encouraged me to put words on a page once I was ready and believed in the value of this book from day one. Likewise, my publisher, Marigold Atkey at Daunt Books Publishing, has cared deeply about this book and has held my hand along the emotional rollercoaster of writing it. Ariella and Marigold, thank you for showing me so much kindness and perspicacity over the four years – *four years!* – it's taken me to write this. Also for your patience.

After a year spent searching the internet for stories to help me make sense of what I was facing, and finding very few, it felt important to me that there were more out in the world. Thank you to Sophie Missing, who bought this book for Daunt before she moved on to a new job. I realise a story about a child with a serious illness and a mother in mental crisis wasn't the most commercial proposition. Thank you for giving it, and me, a shot.

Thank you to the team at Daunt – to Dredhëza Maloku, Jimena Gorráez, Becca Calf, Kate Quarry, Marsha Swan and Jonathan Styles – and all the wider teams at Daunt and Faber. Thank you to Anna Morrison for the exceedingly beautiful cover design. Thank you to Amber Garvey at United Agents.

Thank you to the Society of Authors who, in 2022, awarded me their Authors' Foundation grant, which helped to give me that all-important room of my own in which to write, aka childcare.

Thank you to my wonderful friends and early readers who have helped shape this book. In alphabetical order: Sophie Andrews, Ellie Bateman, Ian Bateman, Rosie Birkett, Laura Brooke, Nick Carvell, Boo Darlison, Liz Davies, Robert Drummer, Joe Farley, Holly Jones, Sophie Mathewson, Katharine Rosser and Lily Saltzberg. A big thank you also to Emily Bryce-Perkins for giving me her expert thoughts, and to Ravinder Bhogal for all the love, food and fundraising.

To Olia Hercules: thank you for reading *Lifeblood* cover to cover so early on, and for the bolstering feedback. You bring both heart and intellect to everything you do, through the hardest of times, and I am lucky to call you my friend.

When Vida was diagnosed, loneliness defined our experience. I'd never heard of DBA, let alone knew anyone with it. I no longer have that problem and I am spoilt for new friends who know all about the singular lives we transfusion and transplant parents lead. Some are mentioned in the book by name, others have asked not to be. In alphabetical order, thank you to Zoe Alderson, Georgie Ashmore, Natalie Barb, Al Gilmour, Emily Gordon-Walker, Kathi Leon, Lauren Tedeschi and Clara White for your solidarity, wisdom and insights. You have all made a lonely path much less lonely.

A special mention for the quite incredible Leisa Batkin, chair of Diamond Blackfan Anaemia Syndrome charity, who advocates for our tiny community, commissions vital research, brings newbies into the fold with warmth and reassurance – and holds down an NHS job as well as parenting four kids of her own.

Thank you also to charities Spread a Smile, Beads of Courage and Rays of Sunshine, who helped wile away hours on hospital wards and encouraged dreams of what lay beyond them.

To Mandy Hopkins for her compassion in epic proportions, and for helping me to understand my amygdala! And all the therapists I saw in that first year: thank you, thank you.

To the NHS, thank you for everything, from the very bottom of my once-broken heart. You are this country's most precious asset. Special thanks to: Professor Josu de la Fuente, Dr Jayanthi Alamelu, Dr Leena Karnik, Dr Adam Gassas, Dr Kirsten Lund, Dr Toni Petterson Dr Dania El Tabech, Dr Albert Borg, Dr Andrew Wilkie, Dr Spyros Bakalis, Dr Tessa Homfray.

Thank you to the wonderful BMT coordinators, Kelly Hennessy, Sandrine Bremathas, Jose Cavalcante. To clinical nurse specialists Yvonne Harrington and Aurica Domocos.

To the PHDU crew: Sara, Gretchen, Ayan, Nana, Susan, Zee; to the GUN girls: Ristell, Habiba, Jaynab, Louise, Maricar, Liberty, Chris, Caroline, Lynette, Glaze, MT, and many more. Each of you has taken great care of us and enriched our lives. Special love to Shirlei da Costa, play specialist extraordinaire and an amazing advocate for the children she works with. To psychologist, Becky Armstrong. To dietician, Katie Elwig. To paediatric dentist, Dr Marielle Kabban. And, of course, to our family on Snow Fox ward at the Evelina: Patrick Gallagher, April, Tola, Charlotte, Claire, Joanna, Michelle, Kelly. All of you. So much love.

Last, but certainly not least, to everyone at NHS Blood and Transplant, and all the blood donors out there. Without all of you, our story – and those of countless others – would be very different indeed. Thank you for making your lifeblood someone else's.

Thank you to our family who have rallied and bubbled with us or supported us from afar for five years.

To our parents: I've lost count of the number of times people have remarked on what amazing support we have in you. We will never take it for granted.

To Louise Webb, I really lucked out with you. You have modelled how to get through the unimaginable with grace, strength and wit, and with your formidable spirit intact. Thank you for scooping us up, innumerable times; thank you for loving me like your own; and thank you for giving me another home – literally and metaphorically.

To Caroline Holland, my mum and my original editor, who sees virtually everything I write before anyone else. In so many ways, I wouldn't be here without you. You really got the worst of me in 2019. I'm sorry. Thank you and thank you to my dad, John, for giving me my love of words – because I think that was instrumental to my getting better. I love you both.

And to the four chambers of my heart: Freddie, Vida and Gabriel (I suppose Ernie is the fourth). This is for you.

Glossary

I do not have a medical background and have relied on doctors putting things into layman's terms over the last few years. Here are some of the words that have cropped up a lot, explained as I understand them.

Amniocentesis
A prenatal test most often used to determine whether a foetus has a health condition. It is typically performed between 15–20 weeks of pregnancy by inserting a small needle into the abdominal wall and removing a sample of amniotic fluid on which to perform genetic testing.

Anaemia
When a person's blood contains insufficient red blood cells or haemoglobin to carry oxygen around the body. Anaemia can present for various reasons; this book describes a genetic condition that causes severe anaemia.

Antithymocyte globulin (ATG)
An antibody preparation infused into patients during bone marrow transplant to prevent their immune system from attacking the donor cells. This better enables those cells to become established and to 'engraft' in the recipient's body.

Bone marrow
The soft and spongey tissue at the centre of most bones. Healthy bone marrow produces stem cells, which themselves produce blood cells, which are vital for sustaining life.

Bone marrow cellularity
The percentage of blood-producing cells in someone's bone marrow relative to the amount of fat tissue. A healthy young child's cellularity is generally very high.

Bone marrow transplant (BMT)
A procedure in which a patient's bone marrow is wiped out using chemotherapy before they are infused with donor stem cells.

Chelation
The umbrella term used to refer to treatments that remove iron from a patient's bloodstream. Chelation therapy can take the form of a daily oral medicine, or a pump inserted via subcutaneous injection (subcutaneous is beneath the skin but above the muscle; in the fatty tissue layer).

Chorionic villus sampling (CVS)
A prenatal test for genetic or chromosomal disorders, usually performed earlier than amniocentesis, at 10–13 weeks pregnancy. A small sample of cells from the placenta is removed through the abdominal wall and tested.

***de novo* mutation**
The term used to refer to a genetic condition caused by a mutation that neither parent has passed on. It therefore has come about 'anew' to a family.

Diamond Blackfan Anaemia Syndrome (DBAS)

A congenital bone marrow failure syndrome characterised by red cell aplasia – when the bone marrow does not make sufficient red blood cells. When Vida was diagnosed, it was known as just Diamond Blackfan Anaemia, but it has since been redefined as a syndrome in recognition that it can include a complex family of symptoms beyond anaemia. In this book, I refer to DBA because this is what I knew it as at that time.

Erythrocyte adenosine deaminase (eADA)

An enzyme detected in the blood, elevated levels of which are used as a confirmatory test in the diagnosis of Diamond Blackfan Anaemia.

Ferritin

A blood protein that stores iron and releases it when needed. In transfusion-dependent patients (who do not make their own red blood cells), ferritin typically soars because they are not recycling iron into new blood cells. Checking a patient's ferritin level is an indirect test of whether a patient has iron overload, and a good indication of whether they should start chelation therapy.

Foetal haemoglobin

The protein that transports oxygen from the mother's bloodstream to a foetus. Foetal haemoglobin has a particularly high affinity for oxygen, meaning it transports it very efficiently to the growing baby.

Graft-versus-host disease (GvHD)

A condition brought about by organ transplant in which the donor cells attack the recipient's cells, recognising them to be foreign. It can affect the skin, gastro-intestinal tract, liver, eyes and more, and it can be suffered acutely or chronically following a transplant procedure. In bone marrow transplant, GvHD is one of the major side effects and risk factors.

Hickman line
A long, flexible plastic tube fitted under the skin of the chest wall. The tube then goes into a large vein just above the heart. During hospital admission for bone marrow transplant, a Hickman line is used to give a patient their many intravenous medications; it is also used to take blood and, sometimes, for intravenous nutrition.

High doppler reading
During pregnancy, dopplers measure the blood flow between mother and baby. A high doppler reading can, among other things, indicate a problem with the placenta, or foetal growth restriction.

Hypocellular
In the context of bone marrow, this means that a patient has fewer cells than 'normal' or typical for their age – usually under 30 per cent.

Mosaicism
When cells within the same person have a different genetic composition – i.e. when a person has more than one genetic line. This can lead to genetic disease that does not present in a parent being passed on to a child.

Magnetic Resonance Imaging (MRI)
A medical technique that uses radio waves and magnetic fields to create a detailed picture of the inside of someone's body. For blood transfusion-dependent patients, MRI is used to assess the liver for iron overload, a procedure also known as FerriScan.

Neutrophils
A type of white blood cell, and one of the body's first lines of defence against micro-organisms such as bacteria and viruses. After chemotherapy, during bone marrow transplant a patient becomes 'neutropenic', meaning they have very few neutrophils with which to fight infection.

Pre-Implantation Genetic Diagnosis (PGD)
A genetic test performed on embryos (conceived through IVF) to determine whether they have a genetic condition.

Prophylactic
The medical term used for a preventative approach. For example, prophylactic medications are given not in response to symptoms but pre-emptively.

Reticulocytes
Immature red blood cells that are produced in the bone marrow then released into the bloodstream. A 'retic count' can help to diagnose a blood disorder like DBA, it also identifies whether the bone marrow is responding appropriately to anaemia – if a patient is anaemic, ideally reticulocytes will increase to compensate.

Stem cells
Always in the news but perhaps poorly understood, medics describe these seemingly magical cells as 'undifferentiated', meaning they are able to become different kinds of cell intended for different functions. Stem cells reside in many parts of the body, but in this book I'm talking about hematopoietic stem cells, or those which originate in the bone marrow and go on to become blood cells.

Select Bibliography

Adichie, Chimamanda Ngozi *Notes on Grief* (London: Fourth Estate, 2021)

Boyer, Anne *The Undying: A Meditation on Modern Illness* (London: Allen Lane, 2019)

Cusk, Rachel *A Life's Work* (London: Faber & Faber, 2001)

Didion, Joan *The Year of Magical Thinking* (London: Fourth Estate, 2006)

Ferrante, Elena *My Brilliant Friend*, translated by Ann Goldstein (London: Europa Editions, 2018)

Freeman, Hadley *Good Girls: A Story and Study of Anorexia* (London: Fourth Estate, 2023)

George, Rachel *Nine Pints: A Journey Through the Mysterious, Miraculous World of Blood* (London: Granta, 2019)

Gessen, Masha *Blood Matters: A Journey Along the Genetic Frontier* (London: Granta, 2008)

Hemon, Alexsander, 'The Aquarium', *New Yorker*, 6 June 2011

Lewis, C. S. *A Grief Observed: A Readers' Edition* (London: Faber & Faber, 2015)

Liptrot, Amy *The Outrun* (Edinburgh: Canongate, 2016)

Lott, Tim *The Scent of Dried Roses* (London: Viking, 1996)

Moore, Lorrie *Birds of America: Stories* (London: Faber & Faber, 2010)

Moxham, Jessica *The Cracks that Let the Light In* (London: Endeavour, 2022)

O'Farrell, Maggie *I Am, I Am, I Am: Seventeen Brushes with Death* (London: Tinder Press, 2018)

Oliver, Mary *New and Selected Poems: Volume One* (Boston, MA: Beacon Press, 2004)

Segal, Francesca *Mother Ship* (London: Chatto & Windus, 2019)

Shapiro, Dani *Inheritance: A Memoir of Genealogy, Paternity, and Love* (London: Daunt Books Publishing, 2019)

Smith, Zadie *Intimations: Six Essays* (London: Hamish Hamilton, 2020)

Sontag, Susan *Illness as Metaphor & Aids and its Metaphors* (London: Penguin Modern Classics, 2009)

Stuart-Smith, Sue *The Well-Gardened Mind: Rediscovering Nature in the Modern World* (London: William Collins, 2020)

Winn, Raynor *The Salt Path* (London: Michael Joseph, 2018)

Daunt Books

Founded in 2010, Daunt Books Publishing grew out of Daunt Books, independent booksellers with shops in London and the south of England. We publish the finest writing in English and in translation, from literary fiction – novels and short stories – to narrative non-fiction, including essays and memoirs. Our modern classics list revives authors whose work has unjustly fallen out of print. In 2020 we launched Daunt Books Originals, an imprint for bold and inventive new writing.

www.dauntbookspublishing.co.uk

We ensure all our products comply with GPSR, CE marking, and other applicable EU Directives. Our EU Responsible Person for GPSR product safety compliance is EU Compliance Partner.

EU Responsible Person (EU RP):

EU Compliance Partner

Postal address: Pärnu mnt. 139b – 14, 11317 Tallinn, Estonia

Contact Email: hello@eucompliancepartner.com

Website: www.eucompliancepartner.com

Phone: +33757690241